CONTENTS

INTRODUCTION

This book is for everyone who cares about what children eat. Whether you have children of your own, teach children or you look after children, you need to know what they should be eating so they will achieve great health and peak performance.

How can you get children to eat food that tastes good, does them good and helps them perform better? Children only eat food they like. If they don't like the taste of it, they won't eat it, no matter how nutritious it may be. But that doesn't mean succumbing to a diet of artificially flavoured, highly sweetened, fat-laden processed food, or existing on fast food and 'kiddie's meals'. Children are perfectly capable of appreciating the taste of healthy foods if you know how to present them — and keep on presenting them! You also need to set a good example yourself. Children are more likely to do as you do, not what you say. So, if they see you enjoying healthy meals and taking part in regular activity, they are more likely to do the same. You can't expect them to eat healthily and take regular exercise if they see you eating confectionery and biscuits, watching TV all the time and taking the car everywhere!

Clearly, the earlier you can help them establish good eating and exercise habits, the more likely they will enjoy a lifetime of good health. My two children don't think twice about walking to school every day, cycling to their after-school activities instead of being driven, and snacking on fruit instead of sweets. They have never known anything different and they have seen both of their parents doing the same.

Kids' Food For Fitness explains what active children should be eating and gives you practical suggestions for healthy meals, snacks and drinks. Unlike other books on kids' nutrition, it emphasises the importance of activity and sport. Whether it's playing in the park, learning to swim or taking part in more serious sports, children will perform better by eating and drinking the right foods. I have witnessed the transformation in children's energy levels and physical performance when they kick unhealthy eating habits and start to eat balanced meals. They have more energy, they suffer fewer colds and minor infections, they have clearer skin and brighter eyes and their powers of concentration at school dramatically increase.

Of course, it's not always easy persuading children to eat healthily. It's difficult to combat the pressures of advertising by manufacturers trying to sell you fatty, sugary foods disguised as children's food. Then there's pester power from your own kids to buy foods sporting their favourite cartoon characters and foods that their friends eat. Believe, me I've had it all from my own children!

Everyone hates the thought of wasting food, so it's easy to get into the routine of giving children only those foods you know they will eat. Time pressures also mean that it's easier to reach for packets and jars than making meals from scratch. The trouble is, children end up eating only a small range of foods and may miss out on important nutrients and exciting flavours. Many of my friends complain that they often get stuck for inspiration and are in desperate need of fresh meal-time ideas. Message received! In this book I have put together four weekly menu plans as well as lots of healthy recipes that are easy to prepare. They have all been tested by willing — and hungry — volunteers. Only those that passed the child-approval test have been kept.

Overweight children are becoming increasingly common, with more than 1 million children under 16 officially classed as obese. They need to be encouraged to become more active, spend less time doing sedentary activities and eat more healthily. At the other end of the scale, some children eat very little and cause a lot of concern to their parents. In this book I give suggestions on dealing with over-weight kids, picky eaters and underweight kids. There is also information about eating disorders and what you can do to help someone suspected of having anorexia or bulimia. Prevention is always the ideal, so I have drawn up a checklist on fostering a positive body image in children.

As you will see, *Kids' Food for Fitness* covers a vast range of nutrition and fitness issues relevant to children. I have combined scientific evidence, recommendations from authoritative experts and information from surveys, with practical sense and my own experience as a sports nutritionist and mother. I hope that you will find the book useful and inspirational, and that you and your children will enjoy fabulous food and great health!

Anita

1 KIDS' FOOD AND HEALTH

The food you feed your children will affect their health now and in the future. It also determines their energy levels, their physical performance and their sporting success. Their brains are also hungry for energy and nutrients so a healthy diet is vital for optimising their mental performance, too. Teaching children to enjoy a healthy, varied diet will help them to grow up healthy, fit and full of energy.

Here are just a few of the benefits that your children will get from improving their diet. They will:

- have more energy and zest
- do better in sport and games
- feel brighter and more alert
- concentrate more easily in lessons
- sleep well and wake up feeling refreshed
- have fewer illnesses
- have clearer skin, brighter eyes and shiny hair

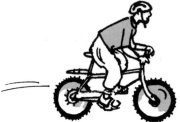

Does it matter what children eat?

Many parents think that it doesn't matter too much what their kids eat, in the belief that their children will soon grow out of unhealthy eating habits. I've seen mums give in to demands for less nutritious food such as sweets and crisps because 'they're skinny so it doesn't matter what they eat' or because 'eating something is better than nothing.' Parents have frequently said to me 'my kids are growing OK

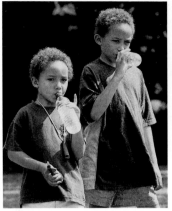

and still running around so their diet can't be too bad.' Wrong on all counts!

The truth is that children's eating habits do not automatically improve as they get older: they nearly always get *worse*. Children continue eating only what they are accustomed to. A bad diet now means a bad diet in five or ten years time. The sooner you start to teach children how to eat healthily, the better. By changing their diet now and helping them to become more active you will increase their chances of enjoying better health now and in the future.

Children need lots of nutrients to make sure they grow and develop properly. The biggest problem with 'junk' food is that it displaces foods that provide important vitamins and minerals. A child who fills up on a chocolate bar has missed out on eating a piece of fresh fruit, or yoghurt or a sandwich — foods which supply a lot more nutrients than sweets.

So, what about their growth? Even if children appear to be growing normally in height that does not mean they are as healthy and fit as they could be. In fact, a child would have to be severely malnourished for his or her growth to suffer, so don't judge children's diets according to whether they are growing. There are many other indicators of poor eating habits. Check the quiz below to find out whether you should change your child's eating habits:

QUESTIONNAIRE
DO YOU NEED TO CHANGE YOUR CHILDREN'S EATING HABITS?

1. Is your child frequently tired and lethargic? ☐

2. Does your child tire easily during physical play or sport? ☐

3. Is your child often pale? ☐

4. Do your child's eyes look dull? ☐

5. Is your child's hair very fine, dry or brittle? ☐

6. Does your child often have difficulty getting out of bed in the morning? □

7. Does your child suffer frequent colds, coughs and infections? □

8. Is your child noticeably fatter than other children of the same age? □

9. Is your child constipated? □

10. Is your child noticeably thinner or smaller than other children of the same age? □

11. Does your child suffer frequent loose bowel movements? □

12. Is your child prone to tummy aches, nausea or sickness? □

13. Does your child often have difficulty concentrating? □

14. Does your child have mood swings? □

15. Is your child often irritable or restless? □

If you ticked 8 or more boxes you definitely need to help your child adopt healthier eating habits

If you ticked between 4 and 8 boxes your child would probably benefit from a healthier diet.

If you ticked fewer than 4 boxes your child's diet may be adequate but is there room for improvement?

This questionnaire is not intended to diagnose or treat any illness or underlying medical condition. You should always check with your doctor if you suspect your child may have an allergy, infection or medical condition.

What are children eating?

Snacking, grazing and eating on the hoof are the norm for many children as they are moving away from regular mealtimes. According to one survey, a quarter of British children eat a breakfast of crisps and sweets before they arrive at school in the morning. One in five children aged between 11 and 16 years miss breakfast altogether. The National Diet and Nutrition Survey of British Schoolchildren revealed that the most commonly eaten foods among 4–18 year olds, eaten by more than 80% of the children, are white bread, crisps, biscuits, potatoes and chocolate bars! Less than half the children ate green leafy vegetables. This survey, the largest of its kind, looked at the diets of 1701 children over seven days and found that:

- Children are eating a mere two portions of fruit and vegetables per day (five portions daily are recommended)
- One in five children eat no fruit at all
- Over 90% of children are eating too much saturated fat
- Most children eat twice the maximum recommended amount of salt
- Half of all girls aged 11–18 years eat diets grossly deficient in iron and magnesium
- Children are eating more than the maximum recommended amount of sugar

It's when these poor eating habits are coupled with inactivity — watching television, playing computer games and getting around by car all the time — that the trouble really begins. Too many calories and too little exercise will cause an unhealthy increase in their body fat.

Why should you change what children eat?

What children eat now influences their future eating habits. If they eat a healthy diet now, and participate in physical activity from an early age, they are more likely to remain healthy and active during adulthood. Children who are used to eating vegetables or walking to school every day (even when it rains) will continue to eat healthy food and see activity as an integral part of their life. Equally, those who graze on a diet of fast foods and salty snacks and spend hours glued to the television are setting themselves up for a lifetime of poor eating habits and inactivity. What's certain is that unhealthy eating and activity habits are harder to undo in later life.

It's also important to realise that the seeds of certain illnesses such as coronary heart disease and diabetes are sown during childhood. Overweight children as young as ten years old are showing signs of artery damage and suffering from high blood pressure. The good news is that changing children's diets and encouraging them to be more active can prevent health problems in the future. *Now* is the time to teach children healthy eating and exercise habits.

So how can I influence children's eating habits?

Children are more likely to do as you do. So, being a good role model will encourage good habits. If children see you enjoying eating healthy foods and taking regular exercise, they are likely to do the same. It's important to realise that attitudes towards food, weight and exercise are established early on. Most eating behaviour is learned.

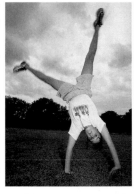

What children see at home makes a big impact on their lifelong eating and exercise habits. Eating a lot of high-fat, salty or sugary foods conditions a child's tastes to those types of food. Unless you make an effort, children will continue to choose bland processed food and reject fresh food such as fruit or vegetables, even though fresh food has stronger flavours. You can't blame them for choosing and eating what they are accustomed to.

Television and advertising

Children are encouraged to eat a poor diet by television advertising. Surveys have found that 95% of the food advertisements on children's prime time television is for foods with high levels of fat, sugar and/or salt (e.g. chocolate, crisps, sweetened breakfast cereals, fast food restaurants), with only very few adverts for healthy foods. This creates a conflict between the types of foods promoted and national dietary recommendations. Moreover, it increases children's 'pester power' as children nag their parents to buy particular products! As there are no controls on the types of food and drinks featured in children's TV, the best action you can take is to set sensible limits on your own children's TV viewing (see Chapter 9, 'Overweight kids', page 77).

How can you combat advertising pressure?

Manufacturers use lots of tricks to persuade you to buy food and drink that is unhealthy for children. Here are the major sneaky promotions used and some suggestions on what you can do to combat them.

CARTOON CHARACTERS ON FOOD PACKAGES

These are designed to grab children's attention and make you buy the product. Many of these types of products are unhealthy and consist of low-quality ingredients.
WHAT YOU CAN DO: *Don't encourage your children to choose which product they want. Look at the label (see page 8). Explain that the food inside is very sugary/fatty/salty.*

ON-PACK PROMOTIONS

Products that contain collectable free gifts or cheap offers for toys and gadgets will appeal to children.
WHAT YOU CAN DO: *Look carefully at what's in the product before you agree to buy it. If it's a product that you would rather not buy, stand firm and steer your children towards healthier choices.*

INTRODUCING LOYALTY

By encouraging token collection for school books, computer equipment, and membership to clubs, or providing interactive websites, manufacturer encourage brand loyalty. This is fine if it's a healthy product, otherwise this ploy pressurises parents to buy products they wouldn't otherwise want for their children.
WHAT YOU CAN DO: *Sorting through tokens is usually tiresome and time-consuming for schools and gives poor value for money.*

A 2001 *Which?* report concluded that such schemes are of questionable benefit. It was calculated that shoppers would need to spend about £220,000 in Tesco, for

TIPS ON CHANGING YOUR FAMILY'S EATING BEHAVIOUR:

- Explain the benefits of eating more healthily (see above). This should be in terms that your children can understand and directly relate to, e.g. having more energy to play football; feeling more refreshed in the morning.

- Put children in control of some of their food choices, e.g. allow them to choose which vegetables to eat; let them suggest a new meal.

- Make some realistic goals (e.g. to eat two pieces of fruit a day; to try a new vegetable; to replace crisps with an apple or a handful of nuts).

- Set up a reward system, e.g. award a star or sticker for each healthy eating behaviour. When, say, 10 stars have been earned, choose a reward (preferably non-food, such as a new toy or a special trip) that has been agreed upon in advance.

- Increase the range of foods in your family's repertoire — try new recipes and offer new snacks (see recipes on pages 131–178).

- Set a good example yourself — don't show reservation in trying new foods.

- Praise children for trying a new food. Even if they don't like it, encourage them to explain why. Try the motto: 'taste before you judge' — it always works with my children who end up eating the lot!

- If a new food or dish is rejected initially, leave it for a while then re-introduce it a week or so later. Children will eventually like healthy foods if they are continually exposed to them.

instance, to get enough vouchers for a computer worth less than £1000 — an unrealistic target for most primary schools. Children would need to buy 50 packets of crips to earn enough tokens for a book worth just £4.00, of which there are only seven on offer — half require five times as many tokens.

NOVELTY VALUE

Children love novelty shapes, 'mini' pack sizes, new textures, and anything that makes a product easy and fun to eat. Great if it's a healthy product — such as fun-sized cheese portions or squeezy yoghurt pots — but many novelty products are high in sugar, fat or salt (as well as being expensive).

WHAT YOU CAN DO: *Make your own healthy novelty food. Chop vegetables or potatoes into fun shapes, serve food in fun dishes, and place healthy snacks like nuts in tiny pots.*

ADDED VITAMINS

By adding extra vitamins to a basically unhealthy product, such as a sugary drink, a sugary processed cereal or a packet of sweets, manufacturers know that parents are more likely to buy it. But this doesn't turn an inherently unhealthy product into a good one. Vitamin-enriched sweets or biscuits are still high in sugar and bad for children's teeth.

WHAT YOU CAN DO: *If you wouldn't have bought the product without vitamins, don't buy it now.*

Looking at the labels

To judge the quality of the food you buy for your children, look at the Nutrition Information panel on food packages. Use the guide below to work out if the food contains unhealthy amounts of fat, sugar or salt (sodium).

AMOUNT PER 100 g (OR PER SERVING IF LARGER THAN 100 g)		
	THIS IS A LOT	THIS IS A LITTLE
Total fat	20 g	3 g
Saturated fat	5 g	1g
Sugar	10 g	3 g
Sodium	0.5 g	0.1 g

What to avoid

ADDITIVES

Additives are supposed to be safe in theory. But they may provoke an allergic reaction or a similar adverse reaction in some children. As additives are found in so many children's foods (up to three-quarters of children's food contains additives, according to a survey by Organix), children could end up eating huge amounts of additives by the time they reach their teens. Sweets, savoury snacks, desserts and snack bars are the worst offenders.

HIDDEN SUGAR

Look out for sucrose, glucose syrup, dextrose, fruit syrup, glucose — they all mean sugar. The main problem with sugar is that it damages children's teeth.

ARTIFICIAL SWEETENERS

Aspartame, acesulphame K and saccharin are common in both 'sugar-free' and ordinary versions of foods and drinks. They may not rot children's teeth but they perpetuate a liking for intense sweetness. Whether they are really safe for children is still a controversial issue.

HYDROGENATED FAT

Check labels for both hydrogenated and partially hydrogenated fats in hard margarines, pastry, pies, cakes, ice cream, desserts, biscuits, chocolate-coated bars, cereal bars and crackers. Solidifying cheap liquid oils produces this type of man-

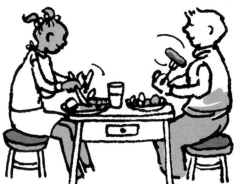

made fat. The problem is that the process also creates trans fats (see page 37), which are even more harmful to health than saturated fats. They increase the levels of 'bad' fats in the blood and reduce levels of 'good fats'.

2 WHAT SHOULD ACTIVE CHILDREN EAT?

All children need to eat a balanced diet to ensure proper growth, good health and physical activity. For active children, eating the right foods is especially important for their performance and recovery after sport. So, how do you set about planning healthy meals for children? This chapter provides a practical guide to meal planning based on the Food Guide Pyramid.

How does the Food Guide Pyramid work?

The Food Guide Pyramid, shown on page 12, is designed to meet the nutritional needs of active children, and makes planning a balanced diet for children easier. It is based on the Health Department Agency's National Food Guide and the US Department of Agriculture's Food Guide Pyramid. The National Food Guide includes only five food groups. This Food Guide Pyramid bumps that number up to the following seven, more finely tuned to the needs of active children: grains, vegetables, fruit, dairy, protein-rich foods, essential fats, sugary and fatty foods. Each group provides some, but not all, of the nutrients and energy children need. The pyramid gives you a visual guide to the proportion of different foods that make up a balanced diet. The lower the layer, the more foods children need from that group for a healthy diet. So, the foods in the bottom layer — grains — should form the bulk of children's diet. The next layer — fruit and vegetables — should be the next most prominent in a child's diet, followed by protein-rich foods and dairy foods. Finally, the foods at the very top of the pyramid — fatty and sugary foods — have a lot of calories from fat and sugars and should be eaten only in small amounts. There are no forbidden foods in the pyramid. Variety and moderation are the most important principles when it comes to putting together a healthy eating plan. Here's how to use the pyramid:

- Include foods from each group in the pyramid each day
- Make sure you include a variety of foods within each group
- Aim to have the recommended number of portions each day
- Check the portion sizes given below

How many portions?

Aim to include the suggested number of portions of each food group each day. Remember, these are guidelines and on some days children may need more or less of a certain food group.

FOOD GROUP	NUMBER OF PORTIONS
Grains	6–8
Vegetables	3
Fruit	2
Dairy	2–3
Protein-rich foods	2–3
Essential fats & oils	1
Sugary and fatty foods	1 or less

How big is a portion?

Of course, the exact amount of each food a child needs varies, depending on their age, size and activity level. In general, younger children need fewer calories than older children so offer them smaller amounts. Their appetites also vary from one day to the next and you'll find that some days they eat much bigger portions than

FOOD PYRAMID

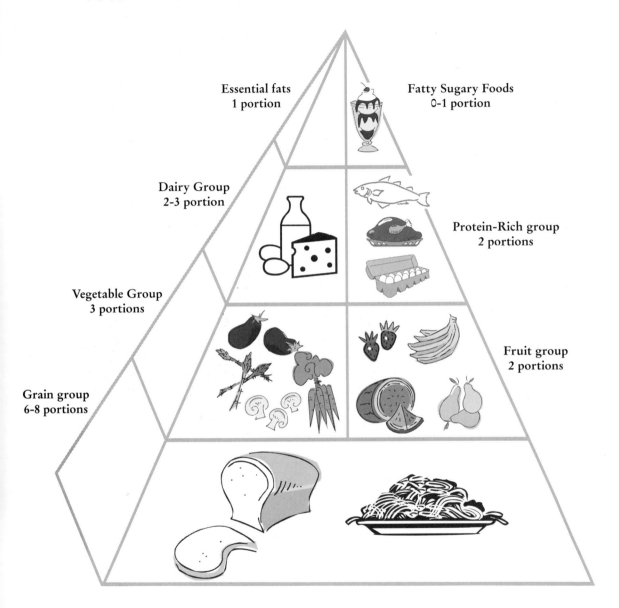

Essential fats
1 portion

Fatty Sugary Foods
0-1 portion

Dairy Group
2-3 portion

Protein-Rich group
2 portions

Vegetable Group
3 portions

Fruit group
2 portions

Grain group
6-8 portions

others. That's fine and, in the main, you should be guided by your children's appetites. Remember it is the overall balance of foods that is most important. The following section gives a guide to suitable portion sizes.

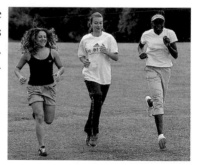

Building the Pyramid

GRAINS AND POTATOES
This group includes bread, pasta, rice, noodles, breakfast cereals, porridge oats, crackers as well as starchy vegetables such as potatoes, sweet potatoes, parsnips and yams. These foods provide complex carbohydrates (starch and fibre) for energy, B vitamins and various minerals including iron. A typical child portion is:

	5–10 YEARS	11–15 YEARS
Bread	1 small slice	1 large slice
Rolls, muffins, bagels	½ large roll	1 large roll
Pasta or rice	3 tablespoons	4 tablespoons
Porridge	3 tablespoons	4 tablespoons
Breakfast cereal	3 tablespoons	4 tablespoons
Potatoes, sweet potatoes, yams	1 small (about the size of an egg)	1 medium (about the size of the child's fist)
Crackers	2	3

Six portions a day can be achieved by:
- A bowl of breakfast cereal
- A slice of toast as a snack
- A jacket potato for lunch
- 2 crackers as a snack
- A pasta or rice dish for supper

FRUIT AND VEGETABLES

Fruit and vegetables are rich in vitamins and minerals, and are also great sources of fibre and phytochemicals, which help protect the body from disease and boost immunity. Offer as many different types of fruit and vegetables in your children's diet as possible. Mix colours — yellow, orange, red, green — so they will get a

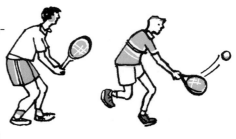

good balance of vitamins and phytochemicals. Try to include at least one green leafy vegetable such as broccoli or cabbage, and one yellow–orange vegetable such as carrots. Offer a variety of fruit too, including yellow–orange fruit such as peaches or satsumas, berries such as strawberries or blackberries and tree fruit such as apples or pears. A typical child portion is:

	5–10 YEARS	11–15 YEARS
Cooked vegetables	2 tablespoons	3 tablespoons
Raw vegetables, e.g. carrot, pepper, cucumber sticks	2 tablespoons	3 tablespoons
Tomatoes	1 medium or 3 cherry tomatoes	2 medium or 6 cherry tomatoes
Apples, pears, oranges, peaches, bananas	1 small piece of fruit	1 medium piece of fruit
Berries e.g. strawberries, blackberries, raspberries	2 tablespoons	3 tablespoons
Small fruit e.g. kiwi fruit, satsumas, plums, apricots	1 piece of fruit	2 pieces of fruit

Five portions a day can be achieved by:

- An apple or kiwi fruit as a snack
- Crudités or vegetable soup for lunch
- Cauliflower cheese and carrots for supper
- Fruit crumble or fruit salad for pudding

DAIRY FOODS

The foods in this group — milk, cheese, yoghurt and fromage frais — are rich in calcium, which is important for children's growing bones. They also provide protein and several of the B vitamins. Full-fat products also contribute fat (mainly saturated) and the fat-soluble vitamins A and D. You can reduce fat easily by switching to reduced fat products, such as semi-skimmed milk or low-fat yoghurt. These are suitable for children over 5 years old. A typical child portion is:

	5–10 YEARS	11–15 YEARS
Milk	I small cup or glass	I medium cup or glass
Yoghurt or fromage frais	I carton	I carton
Hard cheese	2 slices (40 g/1½ oz)	2 slices (40 g/1½ oz)

Two portions a day can be achieved by:
- Breakfast cereal with milk (½ portion)
- Jacket potato with a slice of cheese (½ portion)
- 1 carton of yoghurt (1 portion)

PROTEIN-RICH FOODS

The foods in this group include lean meat, such as beef and lamb (trimmed of fat), chicken, turkey, fish, eggs, beans, lentils, nuts, and soya and quorn meals. They supply protein as well as several vitamins and minerals. Limit meat, sausages, burgers and nuggets to no more than three portions a week because they contain a lot of saturated fat and harmful trans fats (see page 37), not to mention various artificial additives. These fast 'kiddie' foods may appear to be a good solution to teatime dilemmas when you are rushed but they

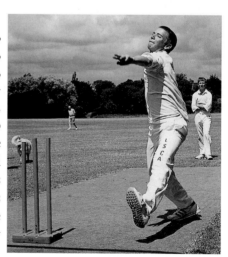

should not be a regular part of your children's menu. If children only ever eat burgers, nuggets and fishfingers, when are they going to learn how to appreciate proper food? The less you rely on these ready-bought fat-laden foods, the better it will be for your children's palates and health.

WHAT ABOUT VEGETARIANS?

Vegetarians get plenty of protein from plant sources, such as beans, lentils and soya products (see page 23). In addition, you may substitute extra dairy foods for one of the portions in this group, as dairy foods are also rich in protein. For example, children may have three portions of dairy foods and one portion of protein-rich foods. However, do not eliminate this group entirely as these foods supply valuable vitamins and minerals not present in dairy foods.

Even if your family are not vegetarian, try to introduce some vegetable protein foods such as beans, lentils and soya products into your children's diet. These foods provide a unique type of fibre that's particularly beneficial for the digestive system, as well as lots of important minerals and phytochemicals not found in animal proteins.

All children should aim to have about half of their portions from non-meat sources.

A typical child portion is:

	5–10 YEARS	11–15 YEARS
Lean meat	1 slice	1–2 slices
Chicken or turkey	2 thin slices	2 medium slices
Fish	Half a fillet	½–1 fillet
Beans and lentils	2 tablespoons	3 tablespoons
Tofu/quorn	½–1 tofu/quorn burger or 2 tablespoons mince	1 tofu/quorn burger or 3 tablespoons mince
Eggs	1 egg	1–2 eggs
Nuts	Small handful	Small handful

Two portions a day can be achieved by:

- Chicken or egg sandwich
- Shepherd's pie made with beef or quorn mince

ESSENTIAL FATS AND OILS

This group includes foods rich in essential oils, the omega-3 and omega-6 oils (see page 35), nuts (walnuts, cashews, almonds, pecans, brazils, pine nuts), seeds (sesame, pumpkin, sunflower), cold-pressed seed and nut oils (flax, pumpkin, walnut, sesame and sunflower), and oily fish (sardines, mackerel, pilchards, trout).

Choose plain, unsalted nuts and avoid those with coatings or flavourings. Lightly toast nuts and seeds under a grill or in a hot oven for a few minutes to bring out their wonderful nutty flavour.

Younger children may find certain nuts and seeds quite hard and may not chew them properly. In this case, ground nuts and seeds (ready-bought or ground in a coffee grinder at home) would be most beneficial. Sprinkle them on salads, muesli or stews. You can even stir them into fruit smoothies.

The nutritional value of nuts, seeds and oils is easily destroyed by heating and by exposure to light and air. So, store in dark bottles in a cool dark place.

A typical child portion is:

	5–10 YEARS	11–15 YEARS
Nuts and seeds	1 tablespoon	1 heaped tablespoon
Nut and seed oils	1 dessertspoon	1 tablespoon
* Oily fish	60 g (2 oz) fish	85 g (3 oz) fish

*Oily fish is the richest source of omega-3 oils so 1–2 portions a week would more than cover a child's needs.

1 portion a day can be achieved by:

- A small handful of nuts or seeds
  OR
- A tablespoon of oil added to a dressing or sauce

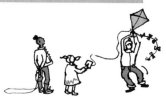

NUT ALLERGIES

Nut allergies seem to be appearing in young children more often than they used to. It is estimated that one in 200 children may be allergic to peanuts. The exact cause is not known but children with nut allergies often have other allergies and other allergy-related conditions such as asthma, hay fever and eczema. A family history of allergy also increases the risk of a child developing a nut allergy. Early signs may include a mild tingling in the mouth or more obvious swelling in the mouth, difficulty in breathing, and swallowing, culminating, occasionally, in anaphylactic shock, which can kill if not dealt with quickly.

The current recommendation is that young children under three years old with a personal or family history of allergy should not be given peanuts in any form. Children with no allergy history can be given peanuts and other nut products after the age of one. Whole nuts should not be given to children under five years old because of the risk of choking.

FATTY AND SUGARY FOODS

This group includes biscuits, cakes, sweets, soft drinks, chocolate and crisps. Aim to limit these foods to once a day because they are high in saturated fat and/or added sugar. They supply relatively large numbers of calories with few, if any, essential nutrients ('empty calories').

The major problem is that if your child eats a lot of these foods, they will have little room left for nutritious foods. Children can develop a 'taste' for intensely sweet, salty processed foods, which takes them even further away from the taste of more natural foods. In other words, sugary fatty foods *displace* healthy foods from a child's diet. Of course, these foods should not be banned from a healthy diet. The idea is to eat them only in moderation, and to regard them as 'extras' or 'treats'.

Children will get all the fats they need from foods in the 'Essential oils' group (nuts, seeds, oils, oily fish), dairy foods and protein-rich foods. Added sugars are, strictly speaking, unnecessary, but can be used sparingly (for example, spreading jam on toast) to enhance the flavour of healthy foods. Encourage your child to enjoy the more natural sweetness of fruit, fruit juice, and dried fruit and fruit desserts. Steer them away from artificially sweetened foods and intensely sugary foods (such as highly sweetened breakfast cereals and fruit squash).

Looking after children's teeth

Eating lots of sugary foods increase the chances of tooth decay, but so do many other foods. Any carbohydrate-containing food that sticks to the teeth will encourage decay, especially if it is eaten frequently throughout the day. Acidic foods and drinks should also be avoided because they cause enamel erosion — literally dissolving the tooth away. There are a number of things you can encourage your children to do to prevent tooth decay and erosion.

- Brush their teeth with a little fluoride toothpaste, ideally after each meal. Aim for a minimum of twice a day, after breakfast and before bed.
- Avoid sweet or sugary foods and drinks between meals.
- Avoid sugary food or drink within an hour of bedtime — water or milk are the only 'safe' drinks.
- Limit 'acidic' drinks, such as soft drinks, squash and fruit juice, to meal times.
- Encourage water between meals, alternatively milk or very diluted fruit juice.
- Avoid sticky foods between meals: sweets, chocolate, biscuits, raisins and other dried fruit and fruit bars. These leave residues on the teeth, increasing the risk of decay. *Note: dried fruit is as potentially harmful to teeth as sweets!*
- If sugary foods or drinks are eaten, then it is better to finish them quickly than eating a packet of sweets or sipping a drink over an hour or more.
- Encourage the drinking of acidic drinks with a straw. This reduces the contact of the drink with the teeth. Sugar-free drinks are not necessarily better for children's teeth as they are quite acidic and can cause dental erosion.

- Have a cube of cheese, plain yoghurt, milk or nuts, at the end of a meal. These foods are 'safe' for teeth. Eating cheese at the end of a meal or as a snack encourages remineralisation of tooth enamel and so helps counteract the harmful effects of sugar and acids.

SNACKS AND DRINKS THAT ARE SAFER FOR TEETH	
SNACKS	DRINKS
Fresh fruit	Water
Yoghurt (preferably unsweetened)	Milk
Cheese (with crackers or bread)	Diluted fruit juice (2 parts water
Toast, plain or with Marmite,	to 1 part juice)
peanut butter or cheese	
Nuts	
Crudités with dips	
Savoury sandwiches	

3 PROTEIN POWER

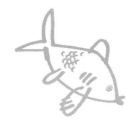

Children need protein to help them grow and develop properly. Protein also makes up your child's muscles, organs, skin and hair. Some protein converts to fuel, supplying energy to exercising muscles. So, do active children need more? Will extra protein benefit children's performance and make them stronger? This chapter explains why protein is needed and how much children should eat. It gives you a guide to planning balanced meals containing the right amounts of protein. If your children do not eat meat, you need to be aware of the nutritional pitfalls. Here you'll find practical advice on vegetarian protein alternatives and how to plan a vegetarian diet.

What happens to protein in the body?

When protein is eaten, it is broken down in the gut into its constituent amino acids. These are absorbed into the bloodstream, taken to the body cells and then re-assembled into new proteins. Here they may be used for:

- Building, maintaining and repairing body cells and organs
- Making hormones and enzymes, which regulate body functions
- Making antibodies, which fight germs and illnesses

Children's body's tissues and organs are by no means fixed — they are constantly being broken down and re-built. This process of repair and renewal takes place much faster in children than adults. That's why you need to make sure they get a regular supply of protein in their diet.

Will extra protein make stronger muscles?

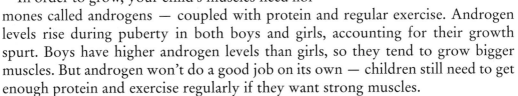

Muscles are made mainly out of protein and water. It's tempting, then, to think that extra protein will help children build bigger and stronger muscles. Or that it will make their muscles work better and improve their performance in sport. But it's not quite that simple.

In order to grow, your child's muscles need hormones called androgens — coupled with protein and regular exercise. Androgen levels rise during puberty in both boys and girls, accounting for their growth spurt. Boys have higher androgen levels than girls, so they tend to grow bigger muscles. But androgen won't do a good job on its own — children still need to get enough protein and exercise regularly if they want strong muscles.

How much protein?

Because children are growing rapidly they need more protein relative to their weight than adults. The reference nutrient intakes for protein published by the Department of Health give a general guideline for boys and girls of different ages. These are given in the table below. Most children need about 1 g per kg body weight (adults need 0.75 g/kg). For example, a 10 year old who weighs 40 kg should eat about 40 g of protein daily. However, the published values do not take account of exercise. Children who are very active or train very hard may need a little more protein.

How to get enough protein

Active children can easily meet their protein needs with a diet that includes two portions from the protein-rich group (lean meat, fish, poultry, eggs, beans, lentils, nuts, tofu and quorn) in the Food Pyramid as well foods from the grains group (bread, pasta, cereals) and dairy group (milk, yoghurt, cheese), which also supply

DAILY PROTEIN REQUIREMENTS OF CHILDREN		
AGE GROUP	BOYS	GIRLS
4–6 years	19.7 g	19.7 g
7–10 years	28.3 g	28.3 g
11–14 years	42.1 g	41.2 g
15–18 years	55.2 g	45.0 g

some protein. Encourage your children to eat a variety of foods from each group. The protein content of various foods is shown in the table overleaf.

Getting enough protein is unlikely to be a problem if children include animal sources of protein (meat, poultry, fish, dairy foods and eggs). If they exclude these foods, you need to make sure they eat a wide variety of plant proteins: beans, lentils, grains, nuts, seeds, soya and quorn (see page 25, box 'Vegetarian diets').

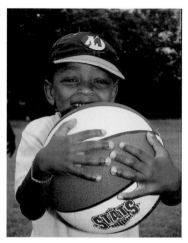

What about vegetarian diets?

To get enough protein from a vegetarian diet, children need to eat a wide variety of plant proteins. This will ensure that they get the right combination of the amino acids essential for growth. There are nine essential amino acids (EAAs), so called because they must be supplied in the diet and cannot be made in the body. Since plant proteins (beans, lentils, soya, grains, nuts) contain smaller amounts of EAAs than animal proteins (meat, poultry, fish, eggs) you need to combine two or more to get the right balance of EAAs. Suitable combinations include:

- Red lentil Bolognese and pasta
- Hummus (chickpea dip) and pitta bread
- Vegetarian chilli with rice

PROTEIN IN VARIOUS FOODS

FOOD	PORTION SIZE	PROTEIN (g)
Meat and Fish		
Lean beef, grilled	1 slice (52 g)	15
Chicken breast, grilled	2 thin slices (65 g)	20
Cod, poached	1 small fillet (85 g)	18
Tuna, canned in brine	½ tin (50 g)	12
Dairy foods		
Cheese, Cheddar	2 slices (40 g)	10
Skimmed milk	1 glass (200 ml)	7
Low-fat yoghurt, fruit	1 carton (150 g)	6
Eggs	1 egg	8
Nuts and seeds		
Nuts and seeds (most varieties)	handful (25 g)	6
Peanut butter	1 tablespoon (20 g)	5
Pulses		
Baked beans	1 small tin (205 g)	10
Red lentils, boiled	3 tablespoons (120 g)	9
Cooked beans, most varieties	3 tablespoons (120 g)	10
Soya and quorn products		
Soya or quorn mince	2 tablespoons (30 g)	13
Tofu burger	1 burger (60 g)	5

- Peanut butter sandwich
- Baked beans on toast
- Tofu or quorn burger in a bun

VEGETARIAN DIETS

A vegetarian diet can be perfectly sound as long as children eat a wide variety of foods from each of the groups in the Food Pyramid. Problems arise only when suitable foods are not substituted for meat. The nutrients most at risk are:

- *Iron* — obtain from wholegrain bread and cereal foods, green leafy vegetables (broccoli, spinach), beans, lentils, nuts, seeds, and iron-fortified breakfast cereals. Offer a vitamin C-rich food or drink (e.g. fruit or fruit juice) at mealtimes as this increases iron absorption.

- *Vitamin B$_{12}$* — obtain from dairy foods or eggs or B$_{12}$-fortified breakfast cereals and soya products.

- *Calcium* — obtain from dairy foods, seeds, calcium-fortified soya products, almonds and oranges.

Sometimes older children — mainly girls — adopt a vegetarian or vegan diet in a misguided attempt to lose weight. If they fail to substitute suitable foods for the meat, or eat only a very limited range of foods, they may be at risk of developing a nutritional deficiency or an eating disorder. If you are concerned, seek advice from a registered dietitian, nutritionist or eating disorder specialist (see Chapter 12, 'Eating disorders').

What about protein supplements?

Protein supplements and meal replacement products containing protein are unnecessary for children. Even the very active should be able to get enough protein from their diet. While such supplements may a have a role to play in the diets of some adult athletes, there is no justification for giving them to children. It is more important that children learn how to plan a balanced diet from ordinary foods and how to get protein from the right food combinations.

4 CARBO-CHARGING

Carbohydrate foods are energy foods and active children need plenty of them not only to fuel their activity but also to support their growth. But it's often difficult to get the balance right between too many sugary foods and not enough grains and fruit. Get it wrong and children may experience flagging energy levels and mood swings. This chapter explains how much carbohydrate they should be eating and helps you to plan a balanced daily diet. It considers which types of carbohydrate are best for health and how to combine different carbohydrates to ensure sustained energy throughout the day.

Why is it needed?

The body turns carbohydrate into glucose, which is then circulated in the blood. Most of the glucose is not needed straight away so it is stored as glycogen in the liver and in the muscles. The main purpose of liver glycogen is to maintain steady blood glucose levels, evening out any peaks and troughs, and keeping a steady supply to fuel the brain. Muscle glycogen, on the other hand, is used to provide fuel for the muscles to do work. So whenever children exercise, muscle glycogen is broken down to supply energy.

How much carbohydrate?

It is recommended that active children obtain around 50–60% of their calories from carbohydrate. For example, a child who needs 2000 calories per day would need to eat 250–300 g of carbohydrate (there are 4 calories per gram of carbohydrate). A good guide is to give children 6–8 portions (depending on their size and energy requirement) from the Grains group in the Food Pyramid: bread, pasta, rice, noodles, breakfast cereals, porridge oats, crackers and starchy vegetables such as potatoes, sweet potatoes, parsnips and yams, as well as two portions from the Fruit group and 2–3 portions from the Dairy group, which also provide some carbohydrate. The exact portion size depends on your child's calorie needs. Generally, older, heavier and more active children need bigger portions. Be guided by their appetite but don't get too prescriptive about the exact amount they should eat. Check the carbohydrate content of various foods in the table on pages 31–2.

This sample menu would be suitable for an active boy aged 7–10 years and provides about 2000 calories. It supplies around 55% calories from carbohydrate, 15–20% from protein and 25–30% from fat.

SAMPLE MENU 7–10 YEAR OLD BOY	
Breakfast	Porridge with raisins and a little honey Orange juice
Snack	Apple and satsuma, water
Lunch	Peanut butter or tuna wholemeal sandwich Carrot and cucumber crudités Yoghurt, grapes Water or diluted fruit juice
Snack (before training)	Cereal bar or bananas, water
Snack (after training)	Dried fruit, water
Supper	Fish Pie, broccoli and carrots Fruit crumble and custard, water

Which types of carbohydrate are best?

The best carbohydrate foods — wholegrain bread, wholegrain cereals, pasta, beans, lentils, potatoes, parsnips, sweet potatoes, fresh fruit, and dried fruit — supply more than just energy. They provide other important nutrients too — B vitamins, iron, zinc, magnesium and fibre — needed for children's growth and development. Make sure that the majority of children's carbohydrate needs come from these unrefined foods.

Highly processed carbohydrate foods, such as white bread, biscuits, sugar, sugary breakfast cereals, sweets and soft drinks should be eaten far less often. The downside is that most of the vital nutrients have been lost during processing. White bread, for example, contains much less fibre, iron, zinc, magnesium and B vitamins than wholemeal bread. Sweets and sugar are virtually devoid of nutrients ('empty calories') so should be kept to a minimum.

The other downside of highly refined foods is that they are 'high glycaemic' foods, or 'fast-releasing' energy foods. This means they are converted into blood glucose rapidly. If children rely on lots of high glycaemic foods for energy, they may develop problems with blood glucose control and you'll certainly notice a change in their energy levels and mood. It is certainly an unsuitable diet for training and sport.

Let's consider what happens when children eat a couple of biscuits or a chocolate bar. The sugars in these foods are broken down into glucose and absorbed very quickly, producing a rapid rise in blood glucose levels. This signals to the pancreas to pump out extra insulin, which in turn causes blood glucose levels to drop rather too quickly. This rapid downswing in blood glucose can make many children feel tired, irritable, hungry and unable to concentrate. A classic case of the 'sugar blues'!

If you do give your child a high glycaemic food, it's a good idea to include a protein-rich food (meat, poultry, fish, eggs, milk, cheese or yoghurt), a high-fat food (oil, butter, nuts, seeds) or a high-fibre food (fruit, vegetables, oats) in the same meal. These are low glycaemic foods ('slow-releasing' foods), which delay the absorption of glucose and so prevent the blood glucose level rising too rapidly, and falling fast.

Some examples of combinations of high glycaemic and low glycaemic foods are listed below.

Carbohydrates and the Glycaemic Index

All types of carbohydrates are digested into simple sugars and then absorbed into the bloodstream. But eventually, they all end up as glucose in the bloodstream. Some carbohydrate foods get there faster than others and this can make a big difference to children's energy levels and physical performance. That's why it's useful to know about the glycaemic index (GI) of foods.

The GI of a carbohydrate food is an indication of how slowly or quickly it pushes up blood glucose levels. Glucose has a score of 100 because it enters the bloodstream faster than all other foods, giving a sharp rise in blood glucose. Foods that are more slowly digested and absorbed such as potatoes, pasta, beans and fruit have a GI value of less than 100 and cause a slower and more sustained rise in glucose levels. The GI of various foods is given in the table on pages 31–2.

The closer the GI value to 100, the faster it is absorbed and turned into blood glucose. Sometimes — for example, after training — a high GI snack is beneficial (see Chapter 7). But in the main, eating lots of high GI snacks is not a good idea, as they will leave children feeling lethargic.

Give children mainly low GI meals and snacks. They are best because they will provide them with long-lasting energy. Of course, they don't need to eat only low GI carbohydrates. By combining a high GI carbohydrate with protein, fat or another carbohydrate with a low GI, you automatically lower the overall GI of the meal. Here are some examples of simple meals that combine a high GI carbohydrate with a low GI food, resulting in an overall lower GI:

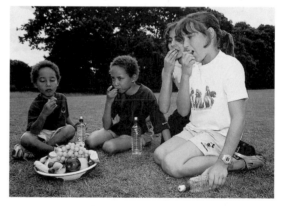

- Jacket potato with cheese
- Pasta with chicken
- Tuna sandwich
- Baked beans on toast
- Biscuit with an apple
- Cornflakes with milk
- Toast with peanut butter
- Cake and yoghurt
- Rice cakes with peanut butter

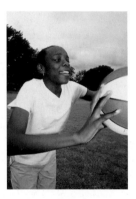
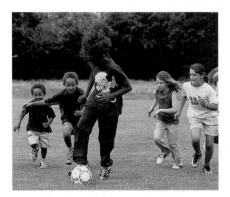

FIBRE

Fibre has three main benefits. Firstly, it helps to keep children's guts healthy, allowing food to pass easily through the body and preventing constipation. Secondly, it helps slow the absorption of glucose into the blood, maintaining steady blood glucose levels and energy levels. And that's vital for active children! Thirdly, foods naturally rich in fibre (wholemeal bread, porridge, fruit, vegetables) are more filling and satisfying. So, children won't get so hungry between meals and ask for sugary snacks. Children can get all the fibre they need from wholegrain bread and cereals, fruit, vegetables, oats, beans, lentils and nuts. There's no need to add bran or lots of bran-enriched cereals.

THE GLYCAEMIC INDEX AND CARBOHYDRATE CONTENT OF FOODS

FOOD	PORTION SIZE	GI	CARBOHYDRATE (g)
Breakfast cereals			
Cornflakes	small bowl (30 g)	84	26
Rice crispies	small bowl (30 g)	82	27
Cheerios	small bowl (30 g)	74	23
Shredded wheat	2 (45 g)	67	31
Weetabix	2 (40 g)	69	30
Porridge (made with water)	small bowl (160 g)	42	14
Muesli	small bowl (50 g)	56	34
Grains/pasta			
Rice — brown	6 tbsp (180 g)	76	58
Rice — white	6 tbsp (180 g)	87	56
Rice — basmati	4 tbsp (60 g)	58	48
Noodles — instant	4 tbsp (230 g cooked)	46	30
Pasta — macaroni	4 tbsp (230 g cooked)	45	43
Spaghetti	4 tbsp (220 g cooked)	41	49
Bread			
White bread	1 large slice (36 g)	70	18
Wholemeal bread	1 large slice (38 g)	69	16
Pizza	1 large slice (115 g)	60	38
Crackers/Crispbreads			
Rice cakes	1 (8 g)	85	6
Biscuits and cakes			
Shortbread	1 (13 g)	64	8
Digestive	1 (15 g)	59	10
Oatmeal	1 (13 g)	55	8
Rich tea	1 (10 g)	55	8
Muffin	1 (68 g)	44	34
Sponge cake	1 slice (60 g)	46	39
Vegetables			
Parsnip	2 tbsp (65 g)	97	8
Potato — jacket	1 average (180 g)	85	22
Potato — boiled, new	7 small (175 g)	62	27
Potato — mashed	4 tbsp (180 g)	70	28
Carrots	2 tbsp (60 g)	49	3
Potato – boiled, old	2 medium (175 g)	56	30
Peas	2 tbsp (70 g)	48	7
Sweetcorn	2 tbsp (85 g)	55	17
Sweet potato	1 medium (130 g)	54	27
Chips	average portion (165 g)	75	59
Pulses			
Baked beans	1 small tin (205 g)	48	31
Chickpeas	4 tbsp (140 g)	33	24
Red kidney beans	4 tbsp (120 g)	27	20
Lentils (red)	4 tbsp (160 g)	26	28

FOOD	PORTION SIZE	GI	CARBOHYDRATE (g)
Fruit			
Pineapple	I slice (80 g)	66	8
Raisins	I tbsp (30 g)	64	21
Apricot	I (40 g)	57	3
Banana	I (100 g)	55	23
Grapes	small bunch (100 g)	46	15
Kiwi fruit	I (68 g)	52	6
Mango	½ (75 g)	55	11
Orange	I (208 g)	44	12
Peach	I (121 g)	42	8
Apple	I (100 g)	38	12
Apricot (dried)	5 (40 g)	31	15
Cherries	small handful (100 g)	22	10
Pear	I (160 g)	38	16
Plum	I (55 g)	39	5
Drinks			
Fanta	375 ml can	68	51
Lucozade	250 ml bottle	95	40
Isostar	250 ml can	70	18
Squash (diluted)	250 ml glass		
	(from 50 ml concentrate)	66	14
Snacks			
Tortillas/corn chips	I bag (50 g)	72	30
Crisps	I packet (30 g)	54	16
Peanuts	small handful (50 g)	14	4
Dairy products			
Ice cream	I scoop (60 g)	61	14
Milk — whole	½ pint (300 ml)	27	14
Milk — skimmed	½ pint (300 ml)	32	15
Yoghurt, fruit (low-fat)	I pot (150 g)	33	27
Confectionery			
Mars bar	I standard (65 g)	68	43
Muesli bar	I (33 g)	61	20
Milk chocolate	I bar (54 g)	49	31
Drinks			
Apple juice	I glass (160 ml)	40	16
Orange juice	I glass (160 ml)	46	14
Sugars			
Glucose	I tsp (5 g)	100	5
Honey	I heaped tsp (17 g)	58	13
Sucrose	I tsp (5 g)	65	5

5 FAT MATTERS

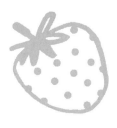

Fat is an important nutrient for children. It not only contributes to their calorie needs but certain types of fats are crucial for their growth and development. This chapter explains which fats are best for children and which ones should be avoided. You'll find a practical guide to the different types of fats and oils to help you untangle the jargon on food labels. Should children restrict their fat intake in order to avoid heart disease? Or will it put them at risk of malnutrition? This chapter tells you how much fat children should be eating and gives some easy ways of cutting down on unwanted fats.

Why is fat needed?

Here are the main reasons why children need fat in their diet.

I. FOR FUEL

Fat supplies energy (calories) that can either be used immediately or stored for future use. In fact, children's fat stores play an important part in fuelling the muscles during many types of physical activity. For example, playing football, running in the playground or swimming all require extra oxygen to make energy. So, fat and carbohydrate (see Chapter 7, 'Eating for action') are broken down to supply the extra energy.

But fat is used to make energy virtually all the time, even while sitting or walking (the only exceptions are during all-out exercise such as sprinting, jumping or throwing). As fat is a very concentrated source of energy (nine calories per gram, compared with four calories for carbohydrate and protein), it can be useful for meeting the energy needs of children who find it difficult to eat enough. On the other hand, those with larger appetites need to take care. Fatty foods (e.g. crisps, biscuits, chocolate) are easy to over-consume as they have little filling-power. See below for guidelines on fat consumption.

2. FOR ABSORBING AND USING VITAMINS

Fat in food helps children's bodies absorb the fat-soluble vitamins A, D, E and K. A fat-free meal (e.g. jacket potato, carrots and peas) would render any fat-soluble vitamins useless. But having a small amount of fat or oil in the meal (e.g. adding margarine or cheese to the potato) helps the body absorb the vitamin A in the carrots. Fats also transport nutrients, such as vitamins and proteins, around the body.

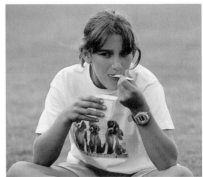

3. FOR GROWTH, DEVELOPMENT AND PEAK HEALTH

Certain kinds of fats and oils are needed for normal growth and development. These are the unsaturated fats, in particular the essential fats (see below). Fats are also an important part of the membranes of all body cells. Without fat, cells simply couldn't exist. But to function at their best, cells need the right ratio of different fats.

4. FOR TASTE AND TEXTURE

Fat contributes to the taste and the texture of many foods and so makes eating more enjoyable. Too little fat and many foods become unpalatable. Too much, of course, can be harmful. It's a question of balance.

What's the difference between saturated and unsaturated fats?

In simple terms, saturated fats are solid at room temperature, whereas unsaturated fats are liquid. *Saturated fats* generally come from animals. For example, the fat in dairy products and meat is high in saturated fats. However, there are two exceptions: coconut and palm (or palm kernel) oils. Despite being vegetable fats, they are both highly saturated. You'll find them in lots of processed foods, such as biscuits, margarine, cakes, desserts, snack bars and pies. If the label simply says 'vegetable fat', chances are it's made from coconut or palm oil. Try to keep saturated fats to a minimum (see guidelines below) because they raise levels of cholesterol in the blood — both in children and adults. There is, in fact, no actual requirement for saturated fats in the diet!

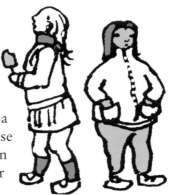

Unsaturated fats generally come from plants. There are two types of unsaturated fats: monounsaturated and polyunsaturated. *Monounsaturated fats* are found in olives, olive oil, rapeseed oil, avocados, nuts and their oils, and seeds and their oils. *Polyunsaturated fats* are found in sunflower, corn and other vegetable oils and oily fish. Both types lower 'bad' cholesterol so they help to reduce the risk of heart disease in later life. But monounsaturated fats have additional health benefits. Unlike polyunsaturated fats, they maintain levels of 'good' cholesterol in the blood while lowering levels of 'bad' cholesterol.

What are the essential fats?

The essential fatty acids (EFAs) are vital for both children's and adults' health. They cannot be made in the body so they must be supplied in the diet. There are two families of EFAs, the omega-3 oils and the omega-6 oils. Oily fish (sardines, salmon, mackerel), pumpkin seeds, walnuts, green leafy vegetables, soya beans, omega-3 enriched eggs, sweet potatoes and certain oils (flaxseed, pumpkin seed, walnut, soya and rapeseed) are the best sources of omega-3s. Most other vegetable oils (e.g. sunflower, safflower, corn), nuts, seeds and whole grains are rich in omega-6s. We need both to be healthy but most of us get too little omega-3s in relation to omega-6s. It's especially important for children to get enough omega-3s. They need them for brain growth and development. These oils also

SOURCES OF FAT		
TYPE OF FAT	FOUND IN	GOOD OR BAD?
Saturated	Meat, burgers, sausages, butter, full-fat milk, cheese, cream, products containing palm or coconut fat ('vegetable fat'), e.g. some margarines.	Bad. It raises blood cholesterol and increases heart disease and cancer risk.
Hydrogenated	Margarine, biscuits, bars, cakes, puddings, other bakery goods.	Bad. Contains trans fats, which increase heart disease and cancer risk.
Polyunsaturated	Vegetable oils (e.g. sunflower, corn), vegetable oil margarine, oily fish, nuts.	Good. Lowers 'bad' cholesterol levels.
Omega-6	Vegetable oils (e.g. sunflower, corn), vegetable oil margarine, nuts, seeds.	Good. Essential for health.
Omega-3	Oily fish, walnuts, pumpkin seeds, soya beans, omega-3 enriched eggs, sweet potatoes.	Excellent. Essential for overall health and brain development, lowers risk of heart attacks and stroke in adulthood, improves sports performance.
Monounsaturated	Olive oil, olives, avocados, nuts, seeds, rapeseed oil.	Good. Lowers 'bad' cholesterol, maintain 'good' cholesterol levels. Reduces heart disease and cancer risk.

help to lower blood fats, and improve oxygen delivery to all body cells. A diet rich in omega-3s will help children's sports performance as they enhance aerobic metabolism.

What is hydrogenated fat?

Hydrogenated fat is made from vegetable oil that has been hardened or hydrogenated. In this process hydrogen is added to the oil to saturate the fatty acid molecules so that it effectively becomes a saturated fat. This new fat is solid at room temperature, rather like butter or lard. Food manufacturers like it because it is cheap, tasteless and less likely to become rancid than other fats. You'll find it in literally thousands of products: cakes, biscuits, pies, pastries, snack bars, cereal bars, crackers, puddings, ice cream and chocolate confectionery.

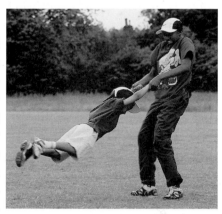

The big problem with hydrogenated fat, apart from being highly saturated, is that it also contains trans fats. These are formed during the hydrogenation process as some of the fat molecules change shape. Trans fats are harmful because they raise 'bad' cholesterol levels as well as lowering 'good' cholesterol levels: a double whammy for pushing up heart disease risk.

Trans fats are not listed on food labels. The only way to avoid them is to check food labels for the words 'hydrogenated fat' or 'partially hydrogenated fat'. It's worrying how many foods specifically targeted at children contain these hydrogenated fats. Be warned.

How much fat should children eat?

Getting the balance right is the key. Taking too much fat out of children's diets can be harmful as they may not get enough calories, fat-soluble vitamins and essential fats, and their growth and development may suffer. Children need slightly more fat relative to their weight and calorie intake compared with an adult. It's important that they get enough calories not only to fuel physical activity but also to support growth.

On the other hand, too much fat will result in excess body fat, reduced physical performance and all the associated risks of obesity (see Chapter 9, 'Overweight kids'). The table below gives the fat content of various foods.

Children aged 5–15 years should get between 25% and 35% of calories from fat. For example, a 10 year old boy who eats 2000 calories a day should get between 55 and 78 g of fat (there are 9 calories in 1 g of fat). The majority of this should come from 'good' fats — that is the unsaturated fats. As a guide, include at least one portion daily from the Essential Fats group (nuts, seeds, seed and nut oils, and oily fish) in the Food Pyramid (see Chapter 2, 'What should active children eat?'). Foods from the Protein-rich group and Dairy group will also supply some fat.

Less than 10% of daily calories should come from saturated fats. The Food Pyramid recommends eating no more than one portion from the sugary and fatty goods group a day.

HOW MUCH FAT?

FOOD	FAT CONTENT
Plain hamburger (110 g)	10 g
Chips (average portion, 110 g)	17 g
2 chocolate digestive biscuits	8 g
1 chocolate bar	12 g
1 packet (30 g) of crisps	10 g
1 chocolate-coated biscuit bar (24 g)	7 g
2 sausages (2 x 20 g)	8 g
1 fairy/cup cake (30 g)	4 g

10 EASY WAYS TO REDUCE FAT
(without missing out on essential nutrients)

1. Serve smaller portions of meat and choose leaner varieties. Trim off any visible fat.

2. Use full-fat dairy products in moderation and swap full-fat milk for semi-skimmed or skimmed milk.

3. Reduce processed and fatty meat products (sausages, salami, pies, burgers).

4. Limit fast food (don't serve these daily): burgers, pizzas with fatty meat toppings, pasties, nuggets, fried chicken pieces, hot dogs.

5. Limit high-fat snack foods: chocolate bars, biscuits, cookies, crisps, muffins, doughnuts, croissants.

6. Serve lower-fat desserts (e.g. yoghurt, frozen yoghurt, fruit crumble, banana custard) in place of high-fat puddings.

7. Keep pastry and pies to a minimum.

8. Provide homemade muffins, cakes and biscuits (see recipes in Chapter 20, 'Kids' snacks'), scones, raisin bagels, English muffins and crumpets in place of traditional cakes and biscuits.

9. Offer fresh fruit, dried fruit, rice cakes or fruit bars in place of biscuits.

10. Serve jacket potatoes or home-made Oven Potato Wedges (see recipe page 162) in place of chips.

6 VITAMINS AND MINERALS

Vitamins and minerals are substances that are needed in tiny amounts to enable your child's body to work properly and prevent illness.

What do vitamins and minerals do?

There are 13 different vitamins, which support almost every system in the body, including the immune system, the brain and nervous system. Many of them help to convert food into energy and help the body to use carbohydrate, fat and protein. They are also involved in regulating growth, making red blood cells, and protecting the body against harmful free radicals.

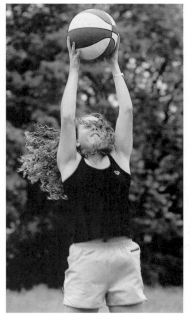

The 15 minerals have mainly structural roles (such as calcium in the teeth and bones) or regulatory roles (e.g. fluid balance, muscle contraction). Iron is one of the most important minerals for active children as it is essential for the production of haemoglobin (the oxygen-carrying pigment in red blood cells). The Vitamins and Minerals Guide below tells you more about the functions and food sources of the key vitamins and minerals.

How to get enough vitamins and minerals

Your children should be able to meet their vitamin and mineral needs by eating the recommended number of portions from each food group in the food pyramid. They should aim for two portions from the fruit group, three portions from the vegetable group, 2–3 portions from the Dairy group, two portions from the Protein-rich group, 6–8 portions from the Grains group and one portion from the Essential Fats group. Vary the choices of foods from each group as much as possible.

WHAT ARE RDAs?

You will find Recommended Daily Amounts (RDAs) listed on food and supplement labels. These are rough estimates of nutrient requirements judged by a group of experts to cover the needs of most people. In the UK, the Department of Health has set RDAs (or, more strictly, Reference Nutrient Intakes, RNIs) for boys and girls in different age categories. The amounts are designed to prevent deficiency symptoms, allow for a little storage, as well as covering differences in needs from one child to the next. They are not targets, rather they are guides to help you check that your child is getting enough nutrients. If you think your child is regularly eating less than the RDAs, you should see a qualified nutritionist or get a GP referral to see a dietitian.

How can you get children to eat more fruit and vegetables?

It is often a struggle to get children to eat the recommended five portions of fruit and vegetables. National surveys have revealed that, on average, children are eating less than two portions a day, a third of the recommended amount! This means that many children are almost certainly missing out on important vitamins and minerals. Here are some ideas for encouraging them to eat more fruit and vegetables:

- Let children plant and harvest their own vegetable garden.

- Get children involved with the shopping — let them choose a new variety of fruit and vegetable (and then, hopefully, eat it!).
- Get children involved with washing, peeling and cutting vegetables.
- Aim to include two different vegetables with the main meal and at least one vegetable with the light meal. Mix colours.
- Aim to include two different fruits, either as snacks or at mealtimes (see following suggestions).
- Establish healthy snack habits, making fresh fruit (whole or cut into bite-sized pieces), carrot, cucumber and pepper matchsticks the norm for at least one snack daily.
- Set a good example yourself. Children are more likely to eat fruit and vegetables if they see you enjoying these foods daily and if there is a plentiful supply in the house.
- Children are more likely to eat small portions of two or three different vegetables than one large portion.
- Top breakfast cereal or yoghurt with chopped fruit e.g. strawberries, bananas, grated apple.
- Crudités (perhaps with hummus, salsa or a cheese dip) make good lunchbox foods (see Chapter 11, 'Eating at school').
- Forget meat and two veg. All-in-one dishes transform vegetables into dishes in their own right: think vegetable curry, vegetable stir-fry, and vegetable chilli.
- Instead of tuna or cheese in jacket potatoes, try ratatouille or sweetcorn.
- The tomato in pasta sauce counts as a portion, but next time, throw in a cupful of chopped broccoli, peppers, courgettes or mushrooms.
- Pass the fruit bowl round after dinner.
- Fruit smoothies and shakes are a delicious way to get a portion or two of fruit. Liquidise strawberries and banana with orange juice.
- Hide vegetables (e.g. carrots, mushrooms, spinach) in Bolognese sauce, in soups, lasagnes, stews, bakes and pies.
- Include salad vegetables in sandwiches or serve on the side.
- For younger children, make vegetables more fun — arrange broccoli and cauliflower as trees on a base of mashed potato; make faces (e.g. use carrots for eyes, baby sweetcorn for a nose, red peppers for the

mouth, broccoli for hair, or whatever else your child likes!).

- Let children decorate their own pizzas with a selection of peppers, mushrooms, tomatoes and pineapple.

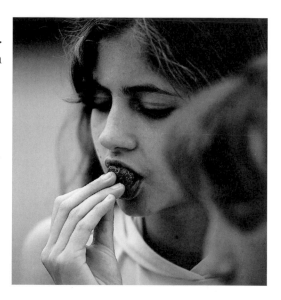

- Instead of sticking to the same vegetables prepared the same way, try new combinations and cooking techniques, e.g. cut carrots, parsnips, swede, courgettes and peppers into chunks, toss in a little olive oil and bake in the oven.

- Add plenty of vegetables to soups (purée or leave chunky), curries and stews.

- Enliven steamed vegetables with a little grated cheese.

- Younger children who refuse most vegetables will often eat 'finger' vegetables, such as sugar-snap peas, baby sweetcorn, green beans, baby carrots, and cherry tomatoes.

- Add a few spoonfuls of frozen peas, sweetcorn or tinned red kidney beans to the saucepan while cooking pasta or rice.

- Fruit, cut into bite-sized pieces, may be more attractive than whole fruit for younger children.

- Children can easily get bored with the same fruit (like apples and bananas) — try exotic fruit (like mangoes, pineapples) or berries (like strawberries or blueberries) at least once a week.

- Use fruit in puddings and desserts. Try baked apples and bananas, fruit mixed with yoghurt, rice pudding topped with fruit, fruit crumbles. See the recipes on pp 163–168.

KEEP THE VITAMINS IN!

- Buy locally-grown produce if you can, ideally from farm shops and local markets.

- Buy British if you have a choice — imported produce is usually harvested under-ripe (before it has developed its full vitamin quota) and will have lost much of its nutritional value during its journey to your supermarket.

- Buy fresh-looking, unblemished, undamaged fruit and vegetables.

- Do not buy fresh produce that is nearing its sell-by date.

- Do not buy ready-cut vegetables, salads or fruit. They will have lost most of their nutritional value by the time you eat them.

- Prepare fruit and vegetables just before you make them into a salad or cook them. From the moment they are chopped they start to lose nutrients.

- Fruit and vegetables should be eaten unpeeled wherever possible because many vitamins and minerals are concentrated just beneath the skin.

- Use frozen food if fresh is not available — it is nutritionally similar.

- Cut into large pieces rather than small; vitamins are lost from cut surfaces.

- Cook vegetables in the minimum amount of water; steaming, microwaving or stir-frying retains the most vitamins.

- When boiling vegetables, add to fast-boiling water and cook as briefly as possible until they are tender-crisp, not soft and mushy.

- Save the cooking water for soups, stocks and sauces.

Guide to Vitamins and Minerals

The following section explains what vitamin and minerals do and how much a 10 year old boy or girl needs to eat to achieve the RDA. Obviously, requirements vary with age, so younger children will usually need slightly less, older children slightly more. (Note: ug=micrograms; mg=milligrams)

VITAMIN A is needed for growth, healthy eyesight, healthy skin, and for colour and night vision.
GET IT FROM: Full fat dairy products, meat, liver, egg yolk, oily fish, margarine, butter. It can also be made from beta-carotene (see below).
HOW MUCH? Get the RDA (500 ug) for vitamin A from a slice (40 g) of liver, or a glass (200 ml) of full-fat milk, two tablespoons (30 g) of margarine and one egg.

BETA-CAROTENE is an antioxidant, which traps and destroys the free radicals that can damage cells and increase cancer risk (see 'Antioxidants' page 54). The body also converts it into vitamin A.
GET IT FROM: Fruit and vegetables, especially orange, red and yellow ones, e.g. carrots, apricots, peppers, tomatoes, mangoes, broccoli, butternut squash, cantaloupe melon, pumpkin.
HOW MUCH? There is no official RDA but you can get the suggested amount (15 mg) from two carrots, half a red pepper and a slice of cantaloupe melon.

VITAMIN B$_1$ (Thiamin) releases energy from carbohydrates. It is also needed for a healthy nervous system and digestive system.
GET IT FROM: Wholemeal bread and cereals, beans, lentils, nuts, meat, sunflower seeds.
HOW MUCH? Get the RDA (0.7 mg) from three slices of wholemeal bread and a small handful of brazil nuts or peanuts.

VITAMIN B$_2$ (Riboflavin) releases energy from carbohydrates. It is also vital for healthy skin, eyes and nerves.
GET IT FROM: Milk and dairy products, meat, eggs, soya products.
HOW MUCH? Get the RDA (1.0 mg) from a small bowl of fortified breakfast cereal, a glass of milk and a pot of yoghurt.

VITAMIN B₃ (Niacin) releases energy from carbohydrates. It also promotes healthy skin, nerves and digestion.
GET IT FROM: Meat, nuts, milk and dairy products, eggs, wholegrain cereals.
HOW MUCH? Get the RDA (12 mg) from two slices of chicken, two slices of wholemeal bread and one egg.

VITAMIN B₆ (Pyridoxine) helps the body to use protein, carbohydrate and fat properly. It is essential for red blood cell manufacture and for keeping the immune system working well.
GET IT FROM: Beans, lentils, nuts, eggs, cereals, fish, bananas.
HOW MUCH? Get the RDA (1.0 mg) from a banana, a portion of white fish and a peanut butter sandwich.

FOLIC ACID is needed for the formation of DNA and of the haemoglobin in red blood cells. It protects against heart disease in later life.
GET IT FROM: Green leafy vegetables, yeast extract, beans, lentils, nuts, pulses, citrus fruit.
HOW MUCH? Get the RDA (150 ug) from a bowl of fortified breakfast cereal, a portion of Brussels sprouts and a portion of Marmite spread on toast.

VITAMIN B₁₂ is essential for growth and red blood cell formation.
GET IT FROM: Milk and dairy products, meat, fish, fortified breakfast cereals, soya products and yeast extract.
HOW MUCH? Get the RDA (1.0 ug) from one egg or two thin slices of red meat or two bowls of fortified breakfast cereal.

VITAMIN C is a powerful antioxidant that protects cells from damaging free radicals. It is also needed for the formation of healthy connective tissue, bones, teeth, blood vessels, gums and teeth; it boosts immune function and helps iron absorption.
GET IT FROM: Fruit and vegetables, especially

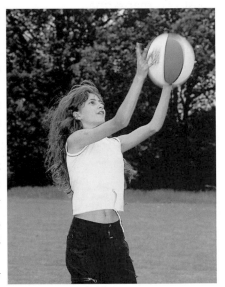

raspberries, blackcurrants, kiwi fruit, oranges, strawberries, peppers, broccoli, cabbage, tomatoes.
HOW MUCH? Get the RDA (30 mg) from one kiwi fruit, or a small glass of orange juice, or two florets of broccoli.

VITAMIN D builds strong bones and teeth. It is needed to absorb calcium and phosphorus.
GET IT FROM: Sunlight (the major source), oily fish, fortified margarine and breakfast cereals, eggs.
HOW MUCH? There is no RDA set for children as the effect of sunlight on the skin allows the body to make enough vitamin D.

VITAMIN E is an antioxidant which helps protects all cells from free radicals and helps prevent heart disease. It also promotes normal cell growth and development.
GET IT FROM: Vegetable oils, oily fish, nuts, seeds, egg yolk, avocado.
HOW MUCH? There is no RDA for children but the Department of Health suggests 5–7 mg is adequate for most adults. There is 5 mg of vitamin E in one tablespoon of sunflower oil or 10 almonds or four florets of broccoli with a slice of wholemeal toast and margarine.

CALCIUM is vital for building strong bones and teeth. It also helps with blood clotting; nerve and muscle function.
GET IT FROM: Milk and dairy products, sardines, dark green leafy vegetables, beans, lentils, brazil nuts, almonds, figs, and sesame seeds.
HOW MUCH? Get the RDA (550 mg) from a glass of milk, a pot of yoghurt and a thick slice of cheese.

DO ACTIVE CHILDREN NEED MORE CALCIUM?
Calcium is a particularly important mineral for growing active children. Along with phosphorus and magnesium it makes up the dense inner part of bones. It's important that children get plenty of calcium in their diet now because their bones are growing rapidly in length, width and shape. If their diet is low in calcium, some calcium will be taken out of the

bones to keep the muscles and nerves functioning properly. This leaves the bones short-changed on calcium, putting them at risk of stress fractures and osteoporosis in later life. Around 90% of the maximum amount of bone minerals is achieved by mid teens. So now is the critical time for building up a good store in their bones.

But it's girls who are the biggest cause for concern. A national survey of British schoolchildren found that many 11–14 year old girls are consuming less than the minimum requirement for calcium, putting them at risk of osteoporosis in adulthood. Many older girls shun dairy products — the richest source of calcium — in the mistaken belief that these foods are 'fattening'. Milk, for example, is substituted by soft drinks, and cheese is viewed as fattening too. While it's not easy to influence older girls' attitudes towards food, here are some ways of encouraging older children to meet their calcium requirement:

- Provide low fat versions of dairy foods, such as skimmed and semi-skimmed milk, low-fat yoghurt, yoghurt drinks, milkshake made with skimmed milk, and low-fat cheeses. Since teenagers tend to drink less milk, encourage them to have more yoghurt and yoghurt drinks. Explain that these are good ways of getting calcium.

- Discourage them from having lots of soft drinks and fizzy drinks. Offer milkshakes made from skimmed milk or low fat yoghurt drinks instead.

- Provide other calcium-rich foods such as canned sardines and salmon (and other tinned fish with edible bones), broccoli, oranges, figs, tofu burgers and almonds.

- Talk to them about the importance of calcium and the risk of brittle bones.

- Be a good role model and consume calcium-rich foods too.

The table below gives the daily calcium requirements for children of different ages and the amounts of various foods providing 200 mg of calcium, roughly one third of the RDA.

DAILY CALCIUM REQUIREMENT (mg)		FOODS CONTAINING 200 mg CALCIUM	
4–6 years (boys and girls)	450	Milk	1 glass (170 ml)
7–10 years (boys and girls)	550	Milkshake	1 glass (180 ml)
11–14 years (boys)	1000	Cheddar cheese	1 slice (25 g)
11–14 years (girls)	800	Yoghurt	1 carton (130 g)
		Broccoli	10 sprigs (500 g)
		Oranges	3 oranges
		Sesame seeds	2 tbsp (30 g)
		Tinned sardines	1½ (36 g)
		Almonds	50 nuts (83 g)
		Dried figs	4 figs (80 g)
		Pizza	1 slice (105g)
		Tofu	1 slice (40 g)
		Ice cream	2½ scoops (250 g)

IRON is essential for the formation of haemoglobin (the oxygen-carrying pigment) in red blood cells. It is also needed for keeping the immune system working well, producing energy and preventing anaemia.

GET IT FROM: Meat and offal, wholegrain cereals, fortified breakfast cereals, beans, lentils, green leafy vegetables, nuts, sesame and pumpkin seeds.

HOW MUCH? Get the RDA (8.7 mg) from one portion of chilli or mince, or a bowl of fortified cereal and two portions of green leafy vegetables.

DO ACTIVE CHILDREN NEED EXTRA IRON?

Because children and teenagers are growing their need for iron is high. The requirement increases sharply during puberty when children have their growth spurt. Iron is, of course, critical not only to good health but also for physical performance. Iron deficiency causes anaemia, which limits oxygen transport in the blood and impairs physical performance.

But low iron stores—even without anaemia—can cause chronic tiredness, lowered resistence to infection, loss of motivation, reduced mental performance and disturb normal energy production in the muscles. So, getting enough iron in the diet is crucial for children. If you suspect that your child may be anaemic consult your GP for a proper diagnosis before giving him iron supplements.

Studies looking at the diets of active children have found that many older girls and teenagers fail to reach the minimum iron requirement, putting them at risk of anaemia. This may be due to their cutting down on red meat (a rich source of iron), coupled with increased iron losses that occur during menstruation. They need to eat alternative iron sources, such as green leafy vegetables, whole grain cereals and beans. The absorption of iron is increased by consuming a vitamin C-rich food or drink at the same meal. For example, top a breakfast cereal with fruit, add broccoli to a pasta dish, have a glass of orange juice with lunch and tea.

The table below shows the daily iron requirements for children and teenagers and food portions providing 2 mg of iron, roughly one quarter of a 10 years old's RDA.

DAILY IRON REQUIREMENT (mg)		FOODS CONTAINING 2 mg IRON	
4–6 years (boys and girls)	6.1	Liver	½ thin slice (16 g)
7–10 years (boys and girls)	8.7	Beef	2 slices (87 g)
11–14 years (boys)	11.3	Baked beans	2 tbsp (141 g)
11–14 years (girls)	14.8	Eggs	2 eggs
		Broccoli	4 florets (180 g)
		Cashew nuts	1 handful (33 g)
		Wholemeal bread	2 slices (40 g)
		Dried apricots	5 apricots (57 g)
		Lentils	2 tbsp (80 g)

ZINC is needed for growth and cell repair. It helps wounds heal quickly and is an essential part of more than 100 enzymes and hormones. It also keeps the immune system healthy and can help protect against colds.
GET IT FROM: Eggs, wholegrain cereals, meat, nuts and seeds.
HOW MUCH? Get the RDA (7 mg) from a portion of red meat and a handful of nuts or pumpkin seeds.

MAGNESIUM works with calcium to make healthy bones. It also assists in muscle and nerve function, regulating the heart beat and in the formation of healthy cells.
GET IT FROM: Whole grain cereals, fruit, vegetables, milk, nuts and seeds.
HOW MUCH? Get the RDA (200 mg) from a small handful of almonds and three slices of wholemeal bread.

Do active children need more vitamins and minerals?

Active children will need greater amounts of most vitamins and minerals compared to those who do little sport. That's because regular exercise increases the demand for all nutrients involved in energy production, cell repair, muscle function and red blood cell formation. In particular, they will need higher amounts of the B vitamins (which help convert carbohydrate into energy), vitamins C and E (both antioxidants, which protect against the increased number of free radicals produced during exercise) and iron (needed to make extra haemoglobin to carry oxygen around the body).

If children eat extra food to meet their increased calorie needs then, providing they eat the right kinds of food, they should automatically be getting more vitamins and minerals.

Should children take vitamin supplements?

In theory, children should not need supplements if they are eating a well-balanced diet and eating a wide variety of foods. But, in practice, not many children manage to do this. Reliance on fast foods, kids' ready-meals, processed snacks, peer pressure and time pressure make this very difficult to achieve. Add to this the fact that most children do not eat the recommended five portions of fruit and vegetables daily, which means that many children may not be getting optimal intakes of many vitamins and minerals.

A well-formulated children's multivitamin and mineral supplement can help ensure they get enough vitamins and minerals so that their growth, physical and mental development and physical performance will not be impaired.

Of course, a supplement should not take the place of a poor diet but it can give you peace of mind that your child won't be missing out on essential vitamins and minerals. Some scientists believe that the RDAs for children are not appropriate as they are based on preventing deficiency symptoms rather than promoting optimal health.

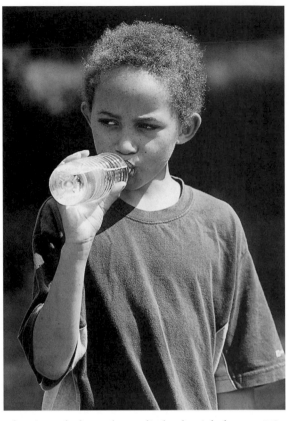

Low intakes of certain vitamins and minerals have been linked with lower IQ, reasoning ability, physical performance, poor attention and behavioural problems. It is possible that supplementation can help correct deficiencies and produce a significant improvement in these aspects of your child. However, extra vitamins and minerals won't make children more brainy or sporty if they are already well nourished.

Make sure you follow the dose directions on the label and don't give children more than one different vitamin or mineral preparation (unless under medical supervision). Keep vitamin supplements well out of young children's reach; they taste and look like sweets!

Phytochemicals

Phytochemicals are plant compounds that have particular health benefits. They include plant pigments (found in coloured fruit and vegetables), and plant hormones (found in grains, beans, lentils, soya products and herbs). Many phytochemicals work as antioxidants (see below), while others influence enzymes (such as those that block cancer agents). They have the following benefits:

- Fight cancer
- Reduce inflammation
- Combat free radicals
- Lower cholesterol
- Reduce heart disease risk
- Boost immunity
- Balance gut bacteria
- Fight harmful bacteria and viruses

For the best protection, encourage children to eat a wide variety of different coloured foods. In general, the more intensely coloured the fruit or vegetable, the greater the concentration of phytochemicals, vitamins and minerals. You can maximise the phytochemical mix by choosing foods from each colour category every day:

- Green — watercress, broccoli, cabbage, rocket, Brussels sprouts, salad leaves, curly kale
- Red/purple — plums, aubergine, cherries, beetroot, red grapes, strawberries, blackberries, blueberries, tomatoes
- Yellow/orange — peaches, apricots, nectarines, oranges, yellow peppers, squash
- White/yellow — onions, garlic, apples, pears, celery
- Brown/green — beans, lentils, bean sprouts, nuts, seeds, tea

Antioxidants

Antioxidants help to protect children's bodies from the effects of free radical damage. They include enzymes (that are made in the body), vitamins (such as beta-carotene, vitamin C, vitamin E), minerals (such as selenium) and phytochemicals. Free radicals are destructive elements which are produced all the time as a normal part of cell processes. In small numbers they are not a problem. But extra free radicals can be generated by pollution, UV sunlight, cigarette smoke and stress. Left unchecked, they can fur up the arteries, and increase the risk of thrombosis, heart disease and cancer. The good news is that antioxidants can neutralise them. And an antioxidant-rich diet may help protect against these conditions and promote faster recovery after exercise.

Antioxidant nutrients are found in fruit and vegetables, seed oils, nuts, whole grains, beans and lentils.

TOP 10 ANTIOXIDANT-RICH FRUIT AND VEGETABLES

Researchers at Tufts University have compiled a league table of fruits and vegetables according to their antioxidant power:

1. Prunes
2. Raisins
3. Blueberries
4. Blackberries
5. Garlic
6. Curly kale
7. Strawberries
8. Raspberries
9. Spinach
10. Brussels sprouts
11. Plums
12. Red peppers
13. Broccoli

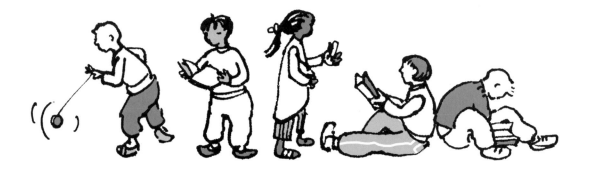

ORGANIC FOOD

Is organic food better for children? Should you consider switching to an organic diet for the whole family? Well, according to a report from the Soil Association in 2001, organic food is most definitely healthier as well as safer.

Perhaps the only drawback is the higher cost of organic food. If you can afford it, just a few organic ingredients will be a step in the right direction. If you can't buy many organic foods, don't worry. It's more important that your child eats plentiful amounts of fresh foods — even if they are non-organic — than skimp on quantities.

Here are 4 reasons for going organic:

1. Organic foods contain the lowest possible amounts of contaminants such as pesticides, antibiotics and nitrates. Although it's a controversial area, there is evidence that the 'cocktail' effect of pesticide residues over time may cause health problems in the future.

2. Organic food can have higher vitamin C levels, and more minerals such as calcium, iron, potassium, zinc and magnesium.

3. Organic foods undergo minimal processing. That means they contain no hydrogenated fats, artificial additives, preservatives or genetically modified organisms (GMOs).

4. Certain organic foods taste better and have more flavour.

GOING ORGANIC

- Buy fruit and vegetables in season when they are cheaper.
- Identify your family's six most frequently eaten foods and try to find organic equivalents.
- Start with salads, fruit and vegetables — of all the food groups, these have the highest pesticide residues so buying organic is the best way to avoid them.
- Join a local box scheme or visit a farmer's market — they offer the best value.
- Snap up seasonal offers or promotions.

7 EATING FOR ACTION

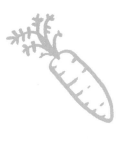

Eating the right foods will help children to perform well in sport. A healthy diet will give them the energy they need to run, swim, cycle and play hard, and reach their sporting potential. What, how much and when they eat will have a big impact on their performance.

This chapter gives you practical guidelines on what children should eat before, during and after exercise. It also deals with the practical problems of fitting meals around training times. There is often little time to eat, especially when training sessions and classes are early in the morning or straight after school. Here you'll find lots of ideas for healthy foods that can be fitted around children's busy schedules. If they are competing or travelling away from home, there's even more reason to ensure they have the right sort of foods and drinks available. Use the checklist and meal ideas in this chapter to make sure they perform at their best.

How much food should my child eat?

Active children need more calories than their less active friends because they need extra energy to fuel their muscles for sport. This extra energy should come mainly from carbohydrate (see Chapter 4, 'Carbo-charging'), with smaller amounts from protein. So plan their diet around foods high in carbohydrate, in the proportions suggested in the Food Pyramid (see Chapter 2, 'What should active children eat?'). They may need slightly larger portions of all the foods in the Food Pyramid compared with their less active friends.

Exactly how much active children should eat is difficult to predict, but the best

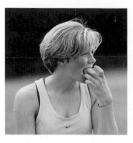

measure really is their appetite. Provided they are not over-weight or underweight (see Chapters 9 and 10), you can safely use their appetite as a guide to portion sizes. Make sure, of course, that they are getting their extra energy from nutritious foods and not simply filling up on sugary, fatty foods.

Be guided, too, by their energy levels. If children are not eating enough, then their energy levels will be persistently low, they will feel lethargic and under-perform at sports. On the other hand, if they appear to have plenty of energy and get-up-and-go, then they are probably eating enough.

It is not realistic to measure the calorie intake of children but you can get a

ENERGY NEEDS OF AVERAGE CHILDREN		
AGE	BOYS (CALORIES)	GIRLS (CALORIES)
4–6 years	1715	1545
7–10 years	1970	1740
11–14 years	2220	1845

CALORIES EXPENDED IN VARIOUS ACTIVITIES	
ACTIVITY	CALORIES IN 30 MINUTES
Cycling (11.2 km/h)	88
Running (12 km/h)	248
Sitting	24
Standing	26
Swimming (crawl, 4.8 km/h)	353
Tennis	125
Walking	88

Values are based on measurements made on adults, scaled down to the body weight of 33 kg, with an added margin of 25%.

rough estimate of whether they are getting it right by checking the values in the first table below. These are the estimated requirements for average children published by the Department of Health. These figures do not take account of regular exercise or sport so you will need to make an allowance for this.

Table 2 lists the estimated calorie expenditure for various activities for a 10 year old child weighing 33 kg. These values are based on measurements made on adults, scaled down to the body weight of a child, with an added margin of 25%. (There are no published values relating to children.) This margin takes account of the relative 'wastefulness' of energy in children compared with adults performing the same activity, due mainly to their lack of coordination. Heavier children will burn slightly more calories than the values in table 2; lighter children will burn less.

What should children eat before training or competition?

Most of the energy needed for exercise is provided by whatever children have eaten several hours or even days before. Carbohydrate in their food will have been converted into glycogen and stored in their muscles and liver (see Chapter 4). If they have eaten the right amount of carbohydrate, they will have high levels of glycogen in their muscles, ready to fuel their activity. If they have not eaten enough carbohydrate, they will have low stocks of glycogen, putting them at risk of early fatigue during exercise.

What they eat just before exercise will not affect their muscle glycogen levels. Rather, it will boost their blood glucose levels, giving them just a little more energy for their activity and possibly postponing fatigue.

Food eaten before exercise needs to:

- Stop children feeling hungry during training
- Be high in carbohydrate
- Provide long-lasting energy
- Be easily digested

Foods with a moderate or low GI (see Chapter 4) are best because they provide sustained energy and will help children keep going longer during exercise. But don't let them eat lots of sugary foods such as sweets and soft drinks just before exercising. This may cause a quick surge of blood glucose followed by a sharp fall, which will leave them feeling lacking in energy and unable to keep going at a good pace.

Avoid high-fat foods too, because they empty from the stomach too slowly. A high-fat snack could make children feel uncomfortable and sick during training. Fats eaten before exercise do not raise blood glucose levels so they will not benefit performance. So what is best? Either a low GI carbohydrate food (e.g. fresh fruit or pasta) or a protein combined with a high GI carbohydrate food (e.g. breakfast cereal with milk) will produce sustained energy. The box below gives some ideas for suitable pre-exercise meals and snacks. It takes a certain amount of trial and error to find out which foods suit an individual child best and exactly how much to eat. Use the box as a guide to the right kinds of foods. Adjust the quantities according to their appetite, how they feel and what they like. It's important that they feel comfortable with the types and amounts of foods. Don't offer anything new before a competition, as it may not agree with them. Drinking is, of course, very important before exercise so make sure children have a glass of water or diluted fruit juice 15–30 minutes before training or competing. See Chapter 8 for more details on drinking.

PRE-EXERCISE SNACKS

Eaten 1–2 hours before exercise; accompany with a drink of water.

- Fresh fruit and glass of milk
- Wholemeal honey sandwich
- Cereal bar or energy bar
- Yoghurt and fresh fruit
- Dried fruit
- Breakfast cereal with milk
- Fruit juice with water (diluted 1:1)
- Crackers with a little cheese
- Homemade muffins and cakes (see recipes on pages 170-175)

PRE-EXERCISE MEALS

Eaten 2–3 hours before exercise; accompany with a drink of water.

- Sandwich/roll filled with tuna, cheese, chicken or peanut butter
- Jacket potato with cheese, tuna or baked beans
- Pasta with tomato-based sauce and fish or beans
- Rice or noodles with chicken or lentils
- Breakfast cereal with milk and banana
- Porridge with raisins
- Lentil/vegetable or chicken soup with wholemeal bread

Timing the pre-exercise meal

The exact timing of the pre-exercise meal may depend on practical constraints, for example, your child's training session or class may be straight after school, leaving very little time to eat. If there is less than one hour between eating and training, give them a light snack (see box 'Pre-exercise snacks'). If they have more than two hours between eating and training, their normal balanced meal will be suitable. This should be based around a carbohydrate food such as bread or potatoes together with a little protein such as chicken or beans, as well as a portion of vegetables and a drink (see box 'Pre-exercise meals').

Eating before an event

If they are competing, you need to make sure that children have access to the right kinds of food. It's usually a good idea to take a supply of food with you as suitable foods and drinks may not be available at the event venue. Children should have their normal meal about

2–3 hours before the event — enough time to digest the food and the stomach to empty. For example, if the event is in the morning, schedule breakfast 2–3 hours before the event start time. Similarly, if the event is in the afternoon, adjust the timing of lunch to 2–3 hours before the event.

Children may feel too nervous or excited to eat on the day of the event. So, offer nutritious drinks (such as diluted fruit juice or sports drinks), milkshakes or light snacks. If they skip meals children may become light-headed or nauseous during the event and will not perform at their best. Here are some simple rules to follow on the day of the event:

- Do not eat or drink anything new
- Stick to familiar foods and drinks
- Take your own foods and drinks wherever possible
- Drink plenty of water or diluted juice before and after the event (see Chapter 8, 'Drinking for action')
- Have high-carbohydrate snacks (see box 'Pre-exercise snacks')
- Avoid high fat foods before the event
- Avoid eating sweets and chocolates during the hour before the event
- Avoid soft drinks (containing more than 6 g sugar/100 ml) an hour before the event
- Encourage children to go to the toilet just before the event

What should children eat during exercise?

If children will be exercising continually for less than 90 minutes, they won't need to eat anything during exercise. They should, however, be encouraged to take regular drink breaks, ideally every 15–20 minutes or whenever there is a suitable break in training or play. Make sure they take a water bottle and keep it within easy reach, for example at the poolside, at the side of the football pitch or by the track (see Chapter 8, 'Drinking for action', page 69).

During an all-day training session or competition, have food and drink available during the short breaks. For example, make opportunities to refuel between swimming heats, tennis games, and gymnastic events. During matches or tournaments lasting more than an hour (e.g. football, cricket or hockey), offer them food and drink during the half-time interval.

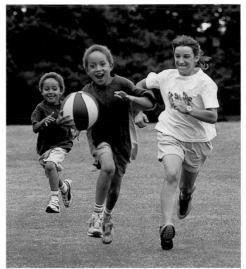

What should they eat? High carbohydrate foods and drinks are the obvious choice as these will help to keep up children's energy, maintain their blood glucose level, delay the onset of fatigue and prevent hypoglycaemia (low blood glucose levels). Similar foods and drinks to those eaten before training or competition are suitable. The important thing is that they are easily digested, high in carbohydrate and low in fat. As you will almost certainly need to take them with you, they should also be non-perishable, portable and quick and easy to eat. Sometimes food is provided at events but you will need to check exactly what will be available beforehand — it may be simply crisps, chocolate bars and soft drinks, all of which are unhelpful for good performance! Check the box below for suitable snacks.

SNACKS FOR SHORT BREAKS DURING TRAINING OR COMPETITION

- Water, diluted fruit juice or sports drinks
- Bananas
- Fresh fruit — grapes, apples, satsumas, pears
- Dried fruit — raisins, apricots, mango
- Crackers and rice cakes with bananas or honey
- Rolls, sandwiches, English muffins, mini-bagels, mini-pancakes
- Fruit, cereal and energy bars

What should children eat after exercise?

After exercise, the first priority is to replenish fluid losses. So give children a drink straight away — water or diluted fruit juice are the best drinks (see Chapter 8, 'Drinking for action').

Children also need to replace the energy they have just used. It's rather like refilling your petrol tank after completing a long journey. And the sooner they eat carbohydrate, the faster they will replenish their energy stores. That's because the body is most efficient at converting carbohydrate into glycogen in the muscles during the first two hours after exercise. In fact, the post-exercise snack or meal is perhaps the most important meal as it determines how fast children will recover before the next training session. Unless they will be eating a meal within half an hour, give them a snack to stave off hunger and promote recovery. The exact amounts you should provide will depend on children's appetite and body size. As a guide, give just enough to alleviate their hunger and keep them going until their mealtime. Studies with adult athletes have shown that 1 g of carbohydrate per kg body weight eaten within two hours of exercise speeds recovery.

So, what are the best foods to eat? High-carbohydrate foods with a moderate or high GI should be included in this recovery snack or meal. They will raise blood

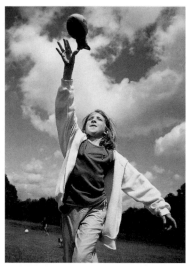

glucose levels fairly rapidly and then be converted rapidly into glycogen in the muscles. Recent studies with adult athletes have found that including a little protein (in a ratio of about 3:1) enhances recovery further. Check the box below for suitable recovery snacks and meals. Unfortunately, most of the snacks on offer in the canteen or vending machines at leisure clubs and sports centres are highly unsuitable. Foods like crisps, chocolate bars, sweets and fizzy drinks will not promote good recovery after exercise. They are little more than concentrated forms of sugar, fat or salt, and actually slow down rehydration. Because they provide a lot of calories too, these foods can take away your child's appetite for healthier foods at the next meal. So what can you

SUITABLE RECOVERY SNACKS

Accompany all snacks with a drink of water or diluted fruit juice.

- Fresh fruit e.g. bananas, grapes, apples

- Dried fruit

- Fruit yoghurt

- Yoghurt drink

- Smoothie (see recipes on pages 176–178)

- Roll or bagel with jam or honey

- Mini-pancakes

- Homemade muffins, bar, biscuits (see recipes on pages 170–175)

- Homemade apple, carrot or fruit cake (see recipes on pages 172–173)

- Homemade milkshake (see recipes on pages 176–178)

SUITABLE RECOVERY MEALS

Accompany all meals with a drink of water or diluted fruit juice and 1–2 portions of vegetables or salad.

- Jacket potatoes with beans, tuna or cheese

- Pasta with tomato sauce and cheese

- Rice with chicken and stir-fried vegetables

- Fish Pie (see recipe on page 133)

- Baked beans on toast

- Fish cakes or bean burgers or falafel with jacket potatoes do? Let your leisure centre know that you are unhappy with the choice of snacks on offer to children, ask other parents and coaches to do the same and suggest that they replace these 'junk' snacks with healthier foods. Any of the suggestions in the box ('Suitable recovery snacks') would be appropriate. As an interim measure, encourage children to take their own drinks and snacks.

Travelling and competing away

When children are travelling to compete away from home, organise their food and drink in advance and take these with you. They may need snacks for the journey so take a supply of suitable foods — use any of the suggestions in the box 'Snacks for eating on the move'. Do not rely on roadside cafes, fast food restaurants, railway or airport catering outlets — healthy choices are often limited at these places. Make sure you take plenty of drinks, in case of delays. Air-conditioned travel in cars, coaches and planes can quickly make children dehydrated.

Try to find out what catering arrangements have been made at the venue. Check the local restaurants and takeaways. Encourage children to choose dishes that are high in carbohydrate, such as pasta, pizza or rice dishes. And warn them against trying anything unfamiliar or unusual — the last thing they need is an upset stomach before the event! When travelling abroad it's best to avoid common food poisoning culprits — chicken, seafood and meat dishes — unless you are sure they have been properly cooked and heated to a high temperature. Be wary of such foods served lukewarm. Check the box below for suitable meals when travelling away.

Remember, too, that children will probably be feeling nervous or apprehensive when travelling away. They may not feel like eating much food. In this case, encourage them to have plenty of nutritious drinks instead, such as fruit juice, smoothies, yoghurt drinks and milkshakes. Pack their favourite foods — of the non-perishable variety — to tempt their appetite.

SNACKS FOR EATING ON THE MOVE

- Sandwiches filled with chicken or tuna or cheese with salad; banana and peanut butter; Marmite

- Rice cakes, oatcakes and wholemeal crackers

- Bottles of water

- Cartons of fruit juice

- Yoghurt drinks

- Individual cheese portions

- Small bags of nuts — peanuts, cashews, almonds

- Fresh fruit — apples, bananas, grapes

- Mini-boxes of raisins

- Fruit bar or liquorice bar

- Sesame snaps

- Prepared vegetable crudités e.g. carrots, peppers, cucumber and celery

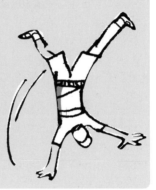

Sometimes it's a case of simply getting them to eat something rather than nothing. If they stop eating they will run down their energy reserves, putting them at a dis-advantage for competition.

SUITABLE RESTAURANT MEALS AND FAST FOODS WHEN TRAVELLING TO AN EVENT

- Simple pasta dishes with tomato sauce
- Rice and stir-fried vegetable dishes
- Pizza with tomato and vegetable toppings
- Simple noodle dishes
- Jacket potatoes with cheese
- Pancakes with syrup

RESTAURANT MEALS AND FAST FOODS TO AVOID

- Burgers and chips
- Chicken nuggets
- Pasta with creamy or oily sauces
- Takeaway curries
- Takeaway kebabs
- Battered fish and chips
- Lukewarm chicken, turkey, meat, fish or seafood dishes
- Hot dogs
- Fried chicken meals

8 DRINKING FOR ACTION

Drinking is just as important as eating. Not only is water essential for keeping children alive and functioning normally, but it also makes a big difference to their physical performance. If children become even mildly dehydrated during exercise they will start to feel unwell and be unable to perform at their best. In fact, early signs of dehydration are easily missed in children, so this chapter tells you what to look out for and how to prevent your child becoming dehydrated during exercise. It also explains which drinks are best for exercising children and whether soft drinks and sports drinks are worthwhile — after all there is a bewildering choice of drinks targeted at children. It's also important to know how much they should drink before and during exercise, so this chapter give some simple guidelines on the amount and timing of drinking around exercise.

Why is drinking important for my child?

Children are much more susceptible to dehydration and overheating than adults for the following reasons:

- They sweat less than adults (sweat help keep the body's temperature stable)
- They cannot cope with very hot conditions as well as adults
- They get hotter during exercise
- They have a greater surface area for their body weight
- They often fail to recognise or respond to feelings of thirst

By the time children are thirsty they will already have lost quite a bit of fluid and may already be dehydrated. Dehydration can set in when they have lost as little as 1 per cent of their body weight. For a 10 year old weighing 34 kg, that would be a mere 0.34 kg. Apart from increased body temperature there are other side-effects:

- Exercise feels much harder
- Heart rate increases more than usual
- May develop cramps, headaches and nausea
- Concentration is reduced
- Ability to perform sports skills drops
- Fatigues sooner and loses stamina

It is impossible for children (and adults!) to per-form at their best when they are dehydrated. You cannot and should not train children to tolerate exercising without drinking. A few sports coaches still restrict fluids during train-ing, in the misguided belief that the human body will eventually adapt to low fluid intakes, or perhaps this is simply to remove the hassle and distraction of drinking itself! However, even if children manage to exercise, they will be per-forming below par. They will also be at risk of developing heat cramps and heat exhaustion.

Dehydration check-up

One of the most reliable tests for dehydration is the 'pee test' — checking the colour, volume and odour of the urine. If it is almost clear or very pale yellow and the child needs to pass urine quite frequently (around once per 1–2 hours), the level of hydration is good. The more intensely coloured it is, the greater the degree of dehydration. Smaller-than-usual volumes of very yellow or gold coloured urine, for example, would indicate that the child is dehydrated and should drink extra water until the urine becomes paler.

WARNING SIGNS OF DEHYDRATION

Children can become dehydrated more easily than adults. Here are some of the signs to look out for.

Early symptoms:

- Unusually lacking in energy
- Fatiguing early during exercise
- Complaining of feeling too hot
- Skin appears flushed and feels clammy
- Passing only small volumes of dark coloured urine
- Nausea

Action: Drink 100–200 ml water or sports drink every 10–15 minutes

Advanced symptoms:

- A bad headache
- Becomes dizzy or light-headed
- Appears disorientated
- Short of breath

Action: Drink 100–200 ml sports drink every 10–15 minutes. Seek professional help.

How much should children drink?

Children need to drink enough fluid to prevent dehydration. On average, children will lose between 350–700 ml of body fluid (equivalent to 0.35–0.7 kg of body weight) during an hour's exercise. If it's hot and humid or they are wearing lots of layers of clothing, they will sweat more and lose even more fluid.

So, children must drink plenty of fluid before, during and after exercise. The exact amount depends on:

- The temperature and humidity of the surroundings — the warmer and higher the humidity, the greater their sweat losses, so they will need to drink more.

- How hard they are exercising — the harder they exercise, the more they sweat, so they will need to drink more.

- How long they are exercising — the longer they exercise, the greater the sweat losses, so they will need to drink accordingly.

- Their size — the bigger they are, the greater the sweat loss, so the more they need to drink.

- Their fitness — the fitter they are, the earlier and more profusely they sweat (it's a sign of good body temperature control) so they will need to drink more than their less fit friends.

Make sure that children are well-hydrated before exercise (see 'Dehydration check-up'). If they are slightly dehydrated at this stage there is a bigger risk of overheating once they start exercising. Encourage them to drink 6–8 cups (1–1½ litres) of fluid during the day and, as a final measure, top up with 150–200 ml (a large glass) of water 45 minutes before exercise.

You can estimate how much fluid children have lost during exercise by weighing them before and after a session. For each 1 kg lost they should drink 1½ litres of fluid. This accounts for the fact that they continue to sweat after exercise and lose more fluid through urine during this time. For example, if a child weighs 0.3 kg less after exercise, he has lost 0.3 litres (300 ml) of fluid. To replace 300 ml of fluid he needs to drink 300 × 1½ = 450 ml of fluid. But don't expect children to drink large volumes after exercising. Divide their drinks into manageable amounts to be taken during and after exercise. A good strategy would be to drink, say, 100 ml at three regular intervals during exercise, then 150 ml afterwards.

Use the following guidelines, in conjunction with the above considerations, to plan your children's drinking strategy:

BEFORE EXERCISE	DURING EXERCISE	AFTER EXERCISE
150–200 ml 45 mins before activity	75–100 ml every 15–20 mins	Drink freely until no longer thirsty, plus an extra glass, or drink 300 ml for every 0.2 kg weight loss

How to fit it all in

Fitting in 6–8 glasses of water a day isn't difficult once children get into the habit of drinking regularly. They could have a glass of water or diluted fruit juice first thing in the morning. Encourage them to have a glass of water, diluted juice or milk (see the list of recommended drinks on page 176) with each meal, a glass between meals, and perhaps a final glass of water last thing at night. It may be more convenient to carry a drinks bottle so that a drink is never far away.

How to make children drink while exercising

- Make drinking more fun with a squeezy bottle or a novelty water bottle.
- Make sure they place the bottle within easy access, e.g. at one end of the pool or by the side of the track, court, gym or pitch.
- Encourage them to take regular sips, ideally every 10–20 mins. This may take practice.
- Tell them not to wait until they are thirsty — plan a drink during the first 20 mins of exercise then at regular intervals during the session, even if they are not thirsty.
- If they are playing in a team sport, work out suitable drink breaks, e.g. half-time during a match, or while listening to the coach during practice sessions.

- If they don't like water, offer a flavoured drink such as diluted fruit juice, dilute squash or a sports drink (see 'What should children drink?').
- Slightly chilling the drink (to around 10 °C) usually encourages children to drink more.

What should children drink?

Plain water is best for most activities lasting less than 90 minutes. It replaces lost fluids rapidly and so makes a perfectly good drink for sport.

But there are two potential problems with drinking water. Firstly, many children are not very keen on drinking water so they simply won't drink enough. Secondly, water tends to quench one's thirst even though the body is still dehydrated.

Encourage water whenever possible, but if your children find it difficult to drink enough water, give them a flavoured drink. Sugar-free squash or ordinary diluted squash are one option. But bear in mind that most brands are laden with additives, including artificial sweeteners, colours and flavourings, which may not be beneficial for your child's health. Organic squashes are better options, although they are more expensive.

Diluted fruit juice (diluted two parts water to one part juice) or isotonic sports drinks are healthier options. Although they probably won't benefit children's performance for activities lasting less than 90 mins, they will encourage them to drink larger volumes of fluid. But a word of caution with commercial sports drinks: in practice, many children find that sports drinks sit 'heavily' in their stomachs. So, you may either dilute the sports drink down with water (if making up from powder, add a little extra water) or alternate sports drinks with water.

If children will be exercising hard and continuously for more than 90 mins, sports drinks containing around 4–6 g of sugars per 100 ml may benefit their performance. This is because the sugars in these drinks help fuel the exercising

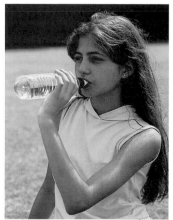

muscles and postpone fatigue. The electrolytes (sodium and potassium) in the drinks are designed to stimulate thirst and make them drink more. Also, at the right dilution (4–6 g/100 ml), these sugars help the body absorb water faster. And the faster you can get water back into the body the better. Always check the sugar content, though. If the drink is too concentrated (more than 6–8 g sugars/100 ml) the drink will stay in the stomach longer (making your child feel uncomfortable) and it will take longer to get absorbed (possibly exacerbating dehydration).

On the downside, sports drinks are relatively expensive. It's cheaper to make your own version by diluting fruit juice (one part juice to one or two parts of water) or organic squash (diluted one part squash to six parts water). Both would also help maintain energy (blood glucose) levels during prolonged exercise.

The most important thing is that children drink enough. Therefore, the taste is important. If they don't like it, they won't drink it! So, experiment with different flavours until you find the ones they like. A little trial and error may be needed to find the best strength drink, too. If it's too concentrated it will sit in their stomachs and make them feel uncomfortable.

CHOOSING THE BEST DRINK FOR EXERCISE

EXERCISE LASTING LESS THAN 90 MINUTES	EXERCISE LASTING MORE THAN 90 MINUTES
Water	Sports drink (4–6 g sugars/100 ml)
Fruit juice diluted 2 parts water to 1 part juice	Fruit juice diluted 1–2 parts water to 1 part juice
Sports drink alternated with water	Squash (ideally organic), diluted 6 parts water to 1 part squash

WHAT CHILDREN SHOULDN'T DRINK!

- Fizzy drinks — the bubbles in fizzy drinks may cause a burning sensation in the mouth, especially if drunk quickly and will certainly stop children from drinking enough fluid. Fizzy drinks can also upset the stomach and make them feel bloated and uncomfortable during exercise.

- Ready-to-drink soft drinks — these are too concentrated in sugar and will tend sit in the stomach too long during exercise. They may make children feel nauseous and uncomfortable.

- Caffeine-containing drinks — these include caffeinated soft drinks, cola, coffee and tea and will dehydrate the body even more. They may also increase the heart rate and cause trembling, as children are more sensitive to caffeine than adults.

SIX WAYS TO KEEP COOL

1. Provide extra water during hot and humid weather.

2. Schedule exercise for the cooler times of the day during hot weather.

3. Schedule regular drink breaks during sessions, ideally in the shade during hot weather.

4. Encourage children to wear loose fitting, natural-fibre clothing during exercise that allows them to sweat freely and permits moisture to evaporate.

5. Let them acclimatise gradually to hot or humid weather conditions — allow two weeks.

6. Make sure they drink extra water 24 hours before a competition.

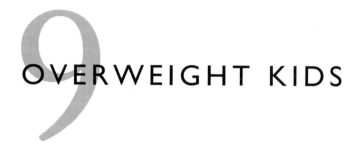

9

OVERWEIGHT KIDS

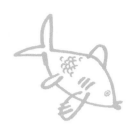

There is little doubt that overweight children are more common nowadays. More than one million children under sixteen are now classified as obese. At just six years old, 9% of British girls are already obese and just over one in five (22%) are overweight, while 11.7% of boys are obese and over one in five (22%) are overweight. By fifteen years old, 17% of girls are obese and 29% overweight, while 16% of boys are obese and 33% are overweight — in other words, roughly half of all fifteen year olds in Britain are obese or overweight, and the figures are rising.

This chapter looks at the reasons why so many children are overweight and offers practical advice on what you can do about it. Clearly, being overweight affects children's health now and in the future. It also affects their physical performance and their self-esteem. Overweight children are more likely to become overweight adults.

Dieting is not the answer. No one wants to see children on fad diets, ruining their health. But at the same time, you cannot sit back and do nothing. This chapter details key strategies to help you deal with children's weight problems.

What are the dangers for children of being overweight?

Although the immediate medical risks of being overweight as a child are small, research has highlighted the following risks for overweight children:

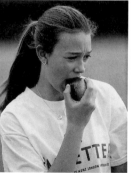

OVERWEIGHT OR OBESE?

Being overweight is defined as having a body mass index (BMI) greater than the norm for that age (between 17.2 and 23.9 BMI, depending on age and gender). Obesity is defined as being significantly over the normal BMI (above 19.2–29.1, depending on age and gender). The BMI is calculated by dividing a child's weight (in kilograms) by the square of their height (in metres). For example, a child weighing 45 kg and measuring 1.4 m would have a BMI of 22.9.

$$\frac{45}{(1.4)} = 22.9$$

BMIs FOR OVERWEIGHT OR OBESE CHILDREN

AGE	OVERWEIGHT		OBESE	
	BOYS	GIRLS	BOYS	GIRLS
5	17.4	17.2	19.3	19.2
7	17.9	17.8	20.6	20.5
10	19.8	19.9	24.0	24.1
12	21.2	21.7	26.0	26.7
15	23.3	23.9	28.3	29.1

- Bone and joint problems — knee, hip and foot problems may develop due to the burden of supporting extra weight
- Breathing problems, particularly at night and during exertion
- High blood pressure
- High blood cholesterol
- Artery damage and increased risk of heart disease in adulthood

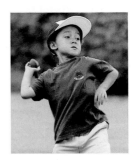

Perhaps the biggest health hazard is that overweight kids are more likely to grow up into overweight adults. And with that comes obesity-related diseases, such as type II diabetes, heart disease and stroke. Most overweight adults were overweight as children. An Australian study of eighteen year olds found that 90% were obese at the age of nine. It also found that being overweight tends to go hand in hand with inactivity and a low level of fitness. What's certain is that poor eating and exercise habits established during childhood are likely to persist. It's more difficult to lose weight or take up sport as an adult than as a child. So, now is the time to act. If children can be encouraged to eat more healthily and take more exercise, they will avoid obesity and more serious problems in adulthood.

FAT PARENTS = FAT KIDS?

Children with overweight parents are more likely to be fat themselves. A study at the Institute of Child Health in London found that seven-year old girls with two overweight parents were 10% heavier than those with parents in the normal weight range. By the age of thirteen, the difference had risen to 20%. A study at Liverpool's Institute of Child Health revealed that children who are more than slightly overweight by the age of seven have a 60% chance of being obese when they are 14–16 years old.

Heart symptoms in obese children

One of the most worrying findings among obese children is the sign of artery damage. In 2001, researchers at the Armand-Trousseau Hospital in Paris found that the arteries of obese children were much stiffer and more damaged than those of normal-weight children. This puts them at greater risk of heart disease and stroke in later life.

How can I tell if a child is overweight?

The easiest way to tell whether children are overweight is by comparing them with their friends of a similar age. Seeing them all in their sports kit or swimming costumes can reveal big differences in body size and body fat.

But, often, children know they are fat — they are told they are by other children. Cruel though this is, if they are teased about their weight at school, it is probably confirmation that they have a weight problem. They may find it hard to take part in sports or other school activities, or may not be able to wear the same clothes as other children. They will begin to feel differently about themselves and may start to feel unhappy.

Sometimes whether a child is overweight is not clear-cut. It is difficult to know whether children are just gearing up for a growth spurt, or if you are projecting your worries about weight onto a perfectly normal child. A stocky or 'well-built' child is most probably fine. But if their tummy hangs over the waistband of their trousers then you may have reason for concern. Height and weight charts only tell you about average children. They don't account for children with different body types, nor do they tell you how much fat an individual child has.

You can perform the pinch test to get a rough idea of how much excess fat a child has. It's not as accurate as skin fold callipers (used for measuring the amount of body fat in adults) but will alert you as to whether you need to take action. Using your thumb and forefinger, see how much excess fat you can pinch just above the hipbones, around the belly button or the lower back. If it's more than an inch then now is the time to talk to them about activity and healthy eating.

Why do children become overweight?

Simply put, children become overweight when there is a mismatch between calorie intake and calorie output. In other words, more calories are consumed from food than are burned during activity. There may be several reasons why this mismatch happens. The key ones are:

- heredity
- overeating
- lack of physical activity

Let's look at each factor a little more closely.

I. HEREDITY

If you look objectively at children's basic body shapes and then compare with their parent's body shapes, you will probably notice a striking similarity. Children's body shapes tend to bear a close resemblance to one of their parents. Just as they inherit blue eyes or brown hair, they can inherit a body type that has a greater tendency to put on weight. This is called the *endomorphic* body type (see box: 'Body types').

Does this mean that you can inherit being overweight? Well, studies have shown that children of two obese parents have an 80% chance of being obese, a 40% chance if only one parent is obese, and yet only a 3% chance if both parents are lean. Studies with identical twins who were adopted by different parents have found that the weights and shapes of the identical twins remained remarkable similar even though they were brought up in different homes.

So, it seems as if you can inherit a greater *tendency* to gain weight. Indeed, scientists have identified several genes that govern appetite and metabolic rate. But — and this is a big but — even if children have inherited a tendency to gain fat, being overweight is by no means inevitable. With a positive attitude, good nutrition habits and regular activity, they can maintain a sensible weight.

BODY TYPES

Anthropologists use three main body type classifications: the ectomorph, the mesomorph and the endomorph. The *ectomorph* tends to be tall, long-limbed and thin. The *mesomorph* tends to naturally muscular with an athletic frame. The *endomorph* has a more rounded frame with a greater tendency to put on excess weight. Few people fit one body type perfectly but everyone has a tendency towards one (or two) body types. So, if a child has mostly endomorphic characteristics, the chances are they have inherited those characteristics from one or both parents.

2. OVEREATING

Many overweight children appear to eat less food than their friends yet they remain overweight. Well, it's not the amount — or volume — of food that matters, it's what they eat and how often they eat.

Look carefully at the kinds of food they eat and how frequently they eat them. Count the number of times they have snack foods such as crisps, chocolate, biscuits, sweets and cakes each day. Do they have regular lunch box treats? What do they eat after school? Do they regularly eat sugary or high-fat snacks in front of the television? Do they rely on fast foods and 'kiddie' meals such as chips, burgers, nuggets and sausages? How often do they have sugar-laden soft drinks, such as squash, cola and other fizzy drinks? The problem with all of these kinds of foods is that they are *dense in calories* — that is, they are full of fat and/or sugar, they contain very little fibre and little water, they have very little 'filling power' and so are very easy to over-eat. Just think how easy and quick it is to eat a few biscuits in front of the TV. They quickly add up to a few hundred calories, which, unless they are used to fuel physical activity, will be stored as fat. Soft drinks are a big culprit. They are high in sugar yet not very filling, so can add a lot of unwanted calories to children's diets. A diet comprising these kinds of foods and drinks is a recipe for disaster.

The solution is not necessarily to ban these foods altogether. Rather, to limit sugary and fatty foods and encourage children to try more nutritious and filling foods. You can instil good eating habits without banning these foods altogether (see below: 'What practical help can I give?').

3. LACK OF PHYSICAL ACTIVITY

Lack of exercise and activity are big problems with many children, whether overweight or not. Combined with unhealthy eating habits, inactivity will certainly lead to overweight. How much time do your children spend sitting — at school, at home, in front of the television or at the computer? If they are sitting in front of the TV or computer, it means that they are not running around and getting exercise. Worse still, television watching lowers the metabolism (the number of calories burned) to barely baseline levels. Researchers have shown that children watching television burn fewer calories than if they were reading or drawing a picture! Television induces an almost trance-like state in children, reducing their energy output to a bare minimum.

How much physical activity do your children do at school? It may be less than you think. There are fewer compulsory sports and PE sessions than ever before. Outdoor break times have been shortened in many schools, the result being that many children get very little exercise during school hours. Do your children get driven to school? A generation ago, most children walked or cycled to school but now traffic congestion and fears for child safety mean that many children are missing out on another opportunity for physical activity. It's common to see children being driven everywhere else, too. Pressures of time mean that many children don't walk or cycle as habit.

GLUED TO THE TELEVISION?

Many experts blame weight problems on too much television. It replaces exercise, significantly lowers the metabolism, encourages unhealthy snacking and increases children's exposure to junk food ads. A four-year study at the Harvard School of Public Health compared the heights and weights of 786 children aged between six and eleven. Those who watched more than five hours of TV a day were more than four times as likely to be overweight as those who watched two hours or less a day.

How should I deal with children's weight problems?

Don't tell children that they should lose weight, even if you are concerned about their weight. Don't punish or scold children — use positive reinforcement. It is important to emphasise feeling healthy and strong. No matter what their size and shape, help them love themselves by praising their strengths and skills. As a parent, reassure them that your love for them is not conditional on how they look or how much they weigh. However, it is important to recognise a weight problem early. Don't sit back and hope that children will 'grow out of it'. The longer a child is overweight, the more difficult it will be to establish a healthy weight. So what's the first step?

For children who are moderately overweight, don't expect them to lose weight as this could compromise their growth and development. Rather, the goal should be weight maintenance rather than weight loss, allowing children to 'grow into' their weight as they get taller. The more slowly this happens, the more likely they will be able to maintain it. Never put children on a 'slimming diet' — they could miss out on essential nutrients and fail to grow normally. Nor should you feed them different meals from the rest of the family, otherwise they will feel more self-conscious about their weight and more likely to rebel against eating healthily. You can help stall their weight gain by concentrating on an overall change towards a healthy lifestyle. Try to approach it in a low-key way, talking about healthy eating rather than 'dieting' and never labelling them as 'fat'. The situation is even more delicate with girls as they are more likely than boys to become obsessed with their weight. Girls, in particular, are bombarded by the media and advertisements with images of slim as beautiful. So it's important that you play down your concerns about your child's or even your own weight.

For children who are very overweight, ask your doctor for advice and a referral to a state registered dietitian. A medically supervised weight loss programme may be suggested, but the emphasis should be on adopting a healthier lifestyle for the long term.

What practical help can I give?

To promote a healthy lifestyle, children should be encouraged to:
- increase their physical activity.
- adopt healthier eating habits.
- reduce the time spent doing sedentary activities.

Think of it as a long-term change rather than a quick fix. Here are some general guidelines:
- Be a role model — they should see that you exercise and eat a balanced diet.
- Encourage the whole family to make healthy food choices and become more active rather than singling out your overweight child.
- Do not impose restrictions on their eating habits that are different from other family members.

- Limit TV viewing and computer time for the whole family. Don't eat in front of the TV.
- Always talk about food in a positive way and discourage talk about weight unless the child brings it up.

How can children be encouraged to be more active?

Make plenty of opportunities for children to be active and give them plenty of support and encouragement. Let them know that exercise is important in everyone's life and should be part of the daily routine. Think of this as a change for the whole family and don't put your focus on your overweight child. Seize daily opportunities to get your family moving and build these into the daily routine. For example:

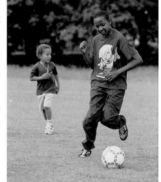

- Walking to and from school and other local places, whenever possible.
- Using the stairs rather than the lift.
- Scheduling a family swim or bike ride at the weekends.

Try to limit the amount of time spent doing passive and sedentary activities, such as watching television and playing computer games. Sedentary activity needs to be balanced with physical activity.

Help children to do more strenuous physical activity. It doesn't mater what it is, provided it lasts for at least 20 minutes and they enjoy it: dancing, cycling, swimming and skating are all great forms of exercise and good fun. Respect your children's individuality and let them make their own choices about exercise as far as possible. For example, let them choose which sport or activity they would like to try — do not force them to take lessons in a particular sport if they dislike it.

Here are some tips for getting them moving:

- Set an example — they will notice whether you lead a physically active lifestyle. Children are more likely to copy what you do than what you say.

- Look for ways to incorporate activity into everything you do, and make this as much fun as possible. Turn activity into games or social activities.
- Walk or cycle with them to and from school — that will benefit both your children and you, and will show them that you are active too.
- *For under-11s*, provide plenty of play equipment at home — hoppers, balls, trampolines, basketball rings, scooters, bikes and skipping ropes.
- Encourage them to enjoy a wide range of sports — football, informal racket games, gymnastics, dance lessons, trampolining and swimming are all suitable for *under-11s*. For *older children*, athletics, roller-skating, hockey, tennis, badminton, netball, jogging, sailing are also suitable.
- They should pick activities that they enjoy — having fun is the key to exercising for life.

How much exercise should children get?

Children from *6–10 years* should do 60 minutes of moderate intensity activity as part of their lifestyle every day. Children aged *11–15* years should do 30–60 minutes of moderate to vigorous activity every day as part of their lifestyle. For both age groups, this recommendation can include everyday activities like walking, unstructured play like ball games, 'chase', and hide and seek, sports activities, and PE. For the *under-11s*, their total activity time can be broken down into several sessions — for example two 15 minute activities in the morning, plus half an hour of activity in the afternoon — it doesn't have to be done in one go. Children aged *11–15 years* should aim for three sessions per week of continuous vigorous activity lasting at least 20 minutes. These could include jogging, swimming, cycling, dancing or football.

How much exercise do children really get?

Children may appear to be doing lots of sport but may not, in fact, be getting much exercise. Observe what they are actually doing during sessions. For example, in cricket and rounders they often spend a lot of time standing or doing very low intensity activity — not enough to build their fitness or manage their weight. If they play team sports such as football, hockey or netball, find out whether they spend most of the time sitting on the bench in reserve or standing in goal. In this case, ask the teacher or coach if they can be moved to other positions or help children select alternative activities that they are better suited to and that they enjoy.

How can children adopt healthier eating habits?

The best that you can do is to offer them information and help. Talk to them about healthy eating, discuss the foods you buy and plan to eat and trust children to make the right choices.

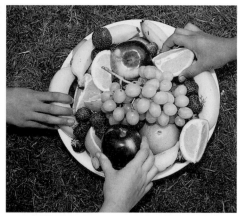

Create healthy habits for the whole family and make mealtimes enjoyable and stress-free. Make sure you do not discuss family conflicts, weight issues or eating habits at the meal table. No foods should be forbidden or labelled in a negative way as this could make children crave 'bad' foods even more and then make them feel guilty when they eat them. Explain that all foods are allowed in a healthy diet, but certain ones should be eaten only occasionally or kept as occasional treats. Never give food as a reward or withhold it as a punishment. Encourage children to eat slowly and to enjoy all foods — even those occasional treats. Discourage secretive eating, over-eating, or eating too fast.

Here are some specific strategies:

- Keep healthy snacks in a place where children can easily get them.
- Eliminate unhealthy foods from your household — remove the temptation for everyone in the family.
- Limit foods high in saturated fats and hydrogenated fats: butter, fried foods, fast foods, biscuits, puddings, chocolate, cakes, crisps and other snacks.

- Use lower-fat cooking methods for family meals.
- Eat foods in the proportions suggested in the Food Pyramid (see Chapter 2), adjusting the portion sizes if necessary.
- Emphasise grains (6–8 portions), fresh fruit (2–4 portions) and vegetables (3–5 portions) in family meals (see the recipes in Chapter 14).
- Offer three nutritious meals a day.
- Offer only healthy snacks (see box below).
- Encourage children to drink water (or diluted fruit juice if necessary) instead of sugary drinks.
- Don't instil that they must eat everything on the plate — encourage them to try everything and to finish when they are full.
- If you need further advice, consult a qualified nutritionist or registered dietitian.

NUTRITIOUS SNACKS

- Wholemeal crackers
- Wholemeal toast with Marmite or honey
- Fresh fruit e.g. apple slices, satsumas, clementines, grapes, strawberries
- Dried fruit e.g. raisins, apricots, apple rings, mango, peaches
- Yoghurt
- Yoghurt drinks
- Toasted nuts e.g. cashews, peanuts, almonds, brazils
- Wholegrain breakfast cereal with milk
- Plain popcorn
- Rice cakes

How can I avoid mealtimes becoming a battleground?

Changing children's eating habits is not easy and requires commitment, resolution and persistence. The sooner you do something about the problem, the better. Provide nutritious meals for everyone — remember not to serve overweight children anything different from the rest of the family. If they refuse certain foods or insist on eating something else, explain that you expect them to try it. Do not give in to unreasonable demands, be resolute and stand firm. If they are hungry, give them only healthy food (fruit, vegetables, grains) not an extra burger or bowl of ice cream. Keep offering those foods they normally refuse and encourage them to try new things. The more you 'give in' to children's demands for less healthy food, the harder and longer it will take to establish healthy eating habits. Remember, children can be very controlling and manipulative with food. It may be hard initially but the eventual rewards will be great.

Should children lose weight for sport?

Children may feel pressurised to lose weight to improve their performance in sport. A lower body fat percentage can improve running speed, jumping ability and performance in most sports. However, children should not be encouraged to attain a lower body fat or weight through dieting or excessive exercise, as this can affect their growth and development. They may not get all the nutrients they need so their health and —ironically — their performance can suffer. Unfortunately, children are often influenced by the successes of thinner teammates or by the remarks of a well-meaning coach.

So what should you do? Children who are a healthy weight for their build should not be encouraged to lose weight. If they are unhappy about their weight, the problem may be one of poor self-esteem or being ill-matched to their sport (see Chapter 12). For example, children with a naturally large build would not be well-matched to sports requiring a thin physique such as long-distance running, ballet, or gymnastics.

If you feel that your children have a genuine weight problem and that losing weight would benefit their performance, health and self-esteem, follow the advice in this chapter and consult with a registered nutritionist or dietitian. Usually an increase in their daily activity level and training intensity, together with a healthier diet, is all that is needed. Allow plenty of time — months rather than weeks — for fat loss. Under professional guidance, children should lose no more than 1–2 kg per month, depending on their age and weight. Weight loss goals must be realistic and achievable for their build and degree of maturity. They should reach this goal at least three or four weeks before competition. This will allow them to compete at their best. You should discourage strict dieting, diuretics, excessive exercise, and use of saunas as weight loss methods as they can be very dangerous for growing children. In the short term, these methods could result in an excessive loss of water, low muscle glycogen stores, fatigue and poor performance. Long-term, they could lead to yo-yo dieting, eating disorders, poor health and impaired development.

How can I discourage television viewing?

- Be selective about what children watch on television. Let them help you plan exactly what they will watch in advance and agree upon a defined time period. Once the time period is up, switch off the television, no matter how much they protest!

- Do not place a TV in children's bedrooms.

- Schedule alternative, preferably physically active activities, in place of television viewing. If you can keep them busy with other activities, they won't have much time left for sitting in front of the television.

- Let the number of hours they have exercised equal the number of hours they are allowed to watch television. If they have done an hour's physical activity during the day, you could allocate an hour's television watching.

- Discourage eating meals or snacks while watching television. Because their mind will be on the television and not on the food, they won't notice when they are full up or not hungry any more.

WEIGHT ISSUES

Many overweight children have low confidence and low self-esteem. Help children develop confidence by praising them for every accomplishment, giving them plenty of opportunities for responsibility, encouraging them to try new skills (e.g. learning to skate or ride a bike) that foster independence and success.

Let children know that they are loved, give them plenty of one-on-one time and physical affection. Let them know that your love for them is not conditional on them losing weight and never suggest that you would love them more if they were to lose weight.

10
UNDERWEIGHT KIDS AND FUSSY EATERS

Some children have small appetites and seem to eat very little, causing enormous worry to their parents. Are they growing properly? Why don't they eat like their friends? Why are they fussy eaters? Trying to feed a fussy eater can be a very frustrating experience that tests a parent's patience and resolve to the limit.

Some children are underweight despite eating normal meals. They struggle to eat enough food to keep their weight up. Active kids who play a lot of sport may burn so much energy that it becomes a problem of how to feed them enough to meet their energy needs. This chapter explores the reasons why some children are underweight, and offers some advice on how to encourage a fussy eater to eat normally. It also gives tips on how active children can maintain or gain weight.

Thin or underweight?

If you are concerned about a child's weight, it's important to work out whether they are clinically underweight or whether they are a thin, yet otherwise perfectly healthy, child. You can reassure yourself that a child is growing normally by asking your doctor to check their height and weight on a standard child growth chart. This will let you know whether their weight is appropriate for their height. If their height is moving parallel to one of the percentile lines and their weight is also moving along in a parallel path, albeit a slightly lower percentile, they are probably fine. However, if their height or weight has fallen off their usual percentile there may be cause for concern. It may be due to recent illness but your doctor will be able to check for any underlying medical condition.

Many underweight children have a naturally very lean build. You can ascertain this by looking at their ankle, knee and wrist joints, and the width of their shoulders, waist and hips. A child with small joints and dimensions, who generally eats well, is probably fine.

Why are some children thin?

There are lots of factors that influence children's weight, shape and size but the key ones responsible for a slim build are:

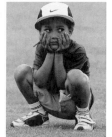

- Heredity
- Under-eating

1. HEREDITY

Children inherit their build and basic body shape from their parents (see Chapter 9, 'Overweight kids', page 77). You'll notice that children with a thin build have a parent, or sometimes a grandparent with a similar build. Compare the basic body shapes of parents and their respective children and you will no doubt see a remarkable resemblance. Thin built people have strong ectomorphic characteristics — that is, narrow shoulders and hips, long lean limbs, with little body fat. Those narrow joints and slender proportions are inherited and will not be affected by what children eat. No amount of food will alter their basic proportions, only the amount of fat they store. If a thin-built child eats extra calories over and above their needs, they will lay down extra fat — not muscle! Clearly, this is not advantageous for health or sport. What is needed is a healthy diet that gives children plenty of energy, while supporting muscle growth and good health.

2. UNDER-EATING

Children who consistently fail to eat enough to meet their energy needs will burn energy from their fat stores and muscle tissue. They may therefore end up carrying very little body fat and will have small muscles.

Do they eat very little at mealtimes? Many young children have a poor appetite, which means they become full after eating relatively little food. See the next section for some practical suggestions on how to feed children with a poor appetite.

Are they fussy eaters? Children often become fussy about food between the ages of one and four years. Choosing and refusing food is one way of asserting their independence. But fussy eating can persist for years, and the longer it is allowed to continue the more difficult it is to get children to accept previously rejected foods. The danger is that fussy eaters could end up not eating enough calories and essential nutrients to support peak health and performance. Again, see *below* for some tips on dealing with fussy eaters.

Do they appear to eat plenty of food but find it a struggle to gain weight? Despite an apparently healthy eating pattern, some children may not be eating enough to meet their high energy needs. They may have a faster-than-average metabolism, which means they burn calories more quickly to keep up their weight and essential functions like heart beat, brain function and digestion. Most children aged 7–10 years need 1740–1970 calories; children aged 11–14 years need 1845–2220 calories. However, if they play a lot of sport and exercise regularly, they may need considerably more — as many as 3000 calories a day (see Chapter 7, 'Eating for action'), and that can be quite hard to achieve. The box below gives tips on increasing children's calorie intake.

Feeding children with small appetites

It can be very frustrating trying to feed children who refuse to eat proper meals. You are probably concerned about them not getting enough calories, becoming malnourished and becoming more vulnerable to illness and infection. The first thing to remember is that children do not voluntarily starve themselves: they are programmed for survival! As long as there is food available, children will make sure they get enough. Secondly, some children are very good at using food to wind up their parents. The more firmly they refuse to finish their plate at mealtimes, the more attention they get. They know that food refusal results in attention (albeit unfavourable) and so a vicious cycle sets up.

So how do you know whether they are eating enough? Think carefully about their total daily intake — it may add up to more than you realise. Do they have snacks between meals? Do they have lots of sugary drinks? Snacks and drinks can amount to a large proportion of children's daily food intake. When children consistently refuse meals, many parents are only too pleased for their child to eat something (even if it's a biscuit) rather than nothing. So it's tempting to give in to demands for snacks.

Now snacks are not necessarily a bad thing, provided they supply nutrients in proportion to their energy content. But if children are filling up on biscuits, soft drinks and crisps they won't be getting the vitamins, minerals and fibre they need. They will be satisfying their hunger with 'empty' calories and have little appetite left for nutritious food at mealtimes.

What's the solution? You need to train children to eat proper meals and nutritious food. Give them no more than two snacks a day — the first between breakfast and lunch and the second between lunch and tea. There should be no extra snacks if they refuse their meal. Suitable snacks could be fresh fruit (such as sliced apples, bananas, grapes or kiwi fruit), cheese, wholemeal crackers, small wholemeal sandwiches or a carton of yoghurt. No matter how much they protest or request unhealthy snacks, stand firm and do not give them any other food. It will be tough at first — no parent wants to 'starve' their child — but after a week or so they will soon get the message that the best thing to do at mealtimes is to eat.

Feeding fussy eaters

Fussy eating is not just confined to the toddler years. Faddy eating habits often persist for many years and, left unchecked, children do not just 'grow out of them'. The earlier you tackle the issue, the better. With older children it just takes more perseverance. Children are entitled to dislike certain foods but some children take this to extremes and are frustratingly fussy. It's not necessary to insist that they clear their plate but you need to persuade them that food is enjoyable and fun. Here are some tips to help you cope with fussy eaters:

- Allow children to help with the shopping and the meal preparation. This will increase their interest in the food, and they will be more likely to eat the meal if they have been involved in making it.

- Encourage the whole family to eat together whenever possible, and always turn off the television at mealtimes.

- Serve children the same food as the rest of the family.

- Serve small portions (even if they seem ridiculously tiny to you) — it's better that they eat a small amount of everything than nothing at all. A big pile of food on the plate can be off-putting for young children.

- Do not discuss eating behaviour, food or family issues at mealtimes. Try to achieve a relaxed atmosphere.

- If they refuse certain foods, explain that you expect them to try it and do not offer an alternative.

- Serve a new food with a food they like.

- Don't keep on telling them to eat up. Children will react to your concern by eating even less and even more slowly.

- Unpopular vegetables can often be disguised — for example, in soup, curries, or pasta sauce.

- If they dislike a particular vegetable, say Brussels sprouts, serve a similar vegetable, say, broccoli (which is also from the Brassica family) or curly kale (which is also a green leafy vegetable), which will provide similar nutrients.

- If a food is rejected, it doesn't mean they will never eat it. Keep re-introducing those foods they reject, say once a week, and don't give up after two or three tries. Remember, it takes up to 8–10 attempts to get a child to eat a new food.

- Allow them to select their own food but from within a limited choice, e.g. 'would you like broccoli or carrots?' rather than 'would you like vegetables?'

- Try not to fuss if they reject a food or refuse to eat.

- Set a sensible time limit (say, 30 mins), after which you take away any uneaten food without a fuss.

- If they don't eat their meal, do not give extra food or snacks between meals (see 'Feeding children with small appetites' above).

- If they are hungry, offer only nutritious food, not a pudding or chocolate bar.

HINTS ON FEEDING UNDERWEIGHT CHILDREN

- Don't fall into the trap of giving in to demands for biscuits and crisps in the belief that 'they need all the calories they can get'. Eating these foods between meals will simply take away children's appetites for more nutritious foods at mealtimes, and perpetuate their taste for those salty, sugary processed foods.

- If they refuse to eat their meal after the allocated time, remove it without fuss and do not offer any other food until the next mealtime. Be consistent and rest assured that they won't become malnourished straight away. This won't be easy but they will soon realise that they only get food at mealtimes.

- Do not 'top them up' with biscuits or sweets after mealtimes. If they are still hungry, offer only nutritious foods, such as fruit, cheese, yoghurt or nuts.

Feeding very active children

For children who struggle to keep up their weight or put on any weight, because they burn a lot of energy in sport, try offering more frequent meals and snacks — six or seven times a day. In fact, snacks are an important part of children's diets. Children have a limited capacity for food, which means they cannot meet their energy demands for growth and activity from three meals only.

The solution is to add on three or four snacks a day, and also make the energy and nutrient content of the food more concentrated. To gain weight, children need to consume more calories than they use for growth and exercise.

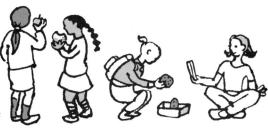

Don't encourage children to cut down the amount of activity or sport they play. Exercise has so many benefits, helping to strengthen their muscles and increase their fitness (see 'Strength training for children').

Here are some suggestions on how to increase the energy intake of children:

- Serve bigger portions, particularly of pasta, potatoes, rice, cereals, dairy products and protein-rich foods.
- Provide three to four nutritious energy-giving snacks between meals — see the box for suggestions.
- Include nutritious drinks, e.g. milk, home-made milkshakes, yoghurt drinks, fruit smoothies and fruit juice.
- Sprinkle grated cheese on vegetables, soups, potatoes, pasta dishes and hotpots.
- Add dried fruit to breakfast cereals, porridge and yoghurt.
- Spread bread, toast or crackers with peanut butter or nut butter.
- Serve vegetables and main courses with a sauce, such as cheese sauce.
- Avoid filling up on stodgy puddings, biscuits and cakes as they supply calories but few essential nutrients (and are usually loaded with saturated or hydrogenated fat).
- Try milk-based or yoghurt-based puddings, e.g. rice pudding, banana custard, fruit crumble with yoghurt, fruit salad with yoghurt or custard, bread pudding, fruit pancakes.

Strength training for children

A strength training or weight training programme, designed to improve total fitness, will improve children's strength, reduce their risk of sports injuries and improve their sports performance. Contrary to the belief that strength training can damage the growth cartilage or stunt their growth, recent studies suggest that it can actually make bones stronger. In fact, there are no reported cases of bone damage in relation to strength training. Children who strength train tend to feel better about themselves as they get stronger, and have higher self-esteem. But strength training is not the same as power lifting, weight lifting or bodybuilding, none of which are recommended for children under 18 years old.

Bulking up should not be a goal of a strength training programme. Children and teenagers should tone their muscles using a light weight (or body weight) and a high number of repetitions, rather than lifting heavy weights. Only after they have

SNACKS FOR WEIGHT GAIN

- Nuts — peanuts, almonds, cashews, brazils, pistachios

- Dried fruit — raisins, sultanas, apricots, dates

- Wholemeal sandwiches with cheese, chicken, ham, tuna, peanut butter or banana

- Yoghurt and fromage frais

- Milk, milkshakes, yoghurt drinks

- Breakfast cereal or porridge with milk and dried fruit

- Cheese — slices, cubes or novelty cheese snacks

- Cheese on toast

- Scones, fruit buns, malt loaf

- Small pancakes

- English muffins, rolls or bagels

- Cereal or breakfast bars (check they contain no hydrogenated fat)

- Bread or toast spread with jam or honey

passed puberty should children consider adding muscle bulk. Younger children should begin with body weight exercises such as push ups and sit ups. More experienced trainees may use free weights and machines.

Sports scientists say that a well-designed strength training programme can bring many fitness benefits for children and can complement an existing training programme. Indeed the American Academy of Paediatrics Committee on Sports Medicine endorses it. Here are some guidelines:

- Children should be properly supervised during training sessions.
- They should use an age-appropriate routine (adult routines are not suitable) — typically 30 second intervals with breaks in-between, with a thorough warm-up and cool-down period.
- Ensure the exercises are performed using proper form and technique.
- Children should start with a relatively light weight and a high number of repetitions.
- No heavy lifts should be included.
- The programme should form part of a total fitness programme.
- The sessions should be varied and fun.

Note: children should complete a medical examination before beginning a strength training programme.

11 EATING AT SCHOOL

Are you happy about what children eat for lunch at school? How can you be sure they are getting a balanced meal that sets them up for the afternoon? How can you influence what they choose to eat at school?

A healthy midday meal helps children to concentrate and participate more fully in lessons. It will provide them with sustained energy to fuel their muscles and their brains. On the other hand, eating the wrong foods will reduce their physical and mental performance.

The healthiest option for eating at school is usually a home-packed lunchbox. At least then you have control over what children eat for lunch and this can make a real difference to their health. It's easy to get stuck in a rut, but altering the contents of their lunchbox throughout the week will make sure they get plenty of variety in their diet, and this can be a great way of introducing children to new foods. This chapter gives you some guidelines on putting together a perfectly balanced lunch and plenty of ideas to make them inspiring and also gives you suggestions for interesting sandwiches and healthy treats.

For children who eat a school lunch, there is less scope for influencing what they eat. However, it may be reassuring to know that the Government introduced minimum nutritional standards for school lunches from 1 April 2001. This chapter gives you the nutritional guidelines for school meals and some hints on encouraging your child to make the best choices.

What are the best foods to eat after school? Whether they play sport or do homework after school, children will need nutritious food to bridge that gap between school and tea. This chapter will give you lots of ideas for healthy snacks.

> **WHAT ARE CHILDREN EATING?**
>
> • Children's favourite items on the school menu are pizza, roast dinner and burgers, according to a survey by school meal caterers.
>
> • One in three children buy sweets, chocolate, soft drinks, crisps and savoury snacks on the way to and from school.
>
> • Children eat chips for lunch between two and three times a week.

Packing a healthy lunch

What you put in children's lunch boxes is critical for balancing their day's nutritional intake. Lunch should supply approximately one third of a child's daily energy needs, as well as one third of their protein, carbohydrate, fibre, vitamin and mineral needs. But getting children to eat a nutritious lunch at school is not always easy. The food you provide has got to look exciting, taste good and be easy to eat. You don't want them returning their lunchbox contents uneaten or, worse, disposing of it in the bin at school. It's easy to fall into the trap of filling it with treats, crisps and chocolate bars to make sure that 'they at least eat something at school'. The problem is that these types of food will quickly become the focus of the meal and other foods will be ignored.

There's also peer pressure to eat the same kind of foods as their friends. Do they insist on having a bag of crisps every day to be like their friends? Again, crisps and savoury snacks can displace healthier foods in the lunchbox and crisp eating will become the norm. Save such food for occasional treats.

Here is a guide to making up a balanced lunchbox menu, based on the food pyramid guide in Chapter 2.

BALANCING THE PERFECT LUNCHBOX:
- A drink (200–300 ml)
- 1–2 portions of fresh or dried fruit
- 1 portion of salad or vegetables (e.g. in a sandwich filling)

- 2–3 portions from the grains group (e.g. either 2–3 slices of bread, 1–2 rolls, 4–6 crackers, small tub of pasta, or a cereal bar)
- 1 portion from the dairy group (e.g. cheese, yoghurt, fromage frais or milk)
- 1 portion from the protein-rich food group (meat, fish, dairy, nuts, beans)

DRINKS

A lunchtime drink will keep children well hydrated and therefore avoid flagging energy levels in the afternoon. Even mild dehydration can causes headaches, fatigue and poor concentration. Remember, children need 6–8 glasses a day (see Chapter 8, 'Drinking for action'). Drinking plenty of fluid is also important to help their kidneys, brain and digestive system work properly.

BEST CHOICES	LESS SUITABLE
Water Milk or milkshake (keep chilled in a thermos) Fruit juice (diluted one part juice, two parts water) Organic fruit cordial (diluted one part cordial ten parts water)	Fizzy drinks (contain too much sugar and too many artificial additives) Fruit drinks, squash and soft drinks (contain too much sugar and too many artificial additives) Sugar-free and 'diet' drinks (contain artificial sweeteners and additives)

FRUIT AND VEGETABLES

A piece of fresh fruit in children's lunchboxes will help make up the daily goal of two portions suggested in the Food Pyramid. All types of fruit and vegetables — including dried and tinned varieties — supply vitamins, minerals and phytochemicals (see Chapter 6, 'Vitamins and minerals'). Fruits that are easy to eat or prepare are best (see the box below). If a whole piece of fruit is unappealing, chop it into pieces or supply a knife (e.g. for apples) or spoon (e.g. for kiwi fruit) to make it easier for them to eat. When my six-year old first took a kiwi fruit with a small knife and spoon to school, her friends were so intrigued, they requested one too!

Small ring-pull tins of fruit in juice and small cartons of fruit purée are also ideal for lunch boxes — look out for them in your supermarket.

Small boxes and bags of dried fruit are also good choices. They are fun to eat and supply good amounts of fibre and various vitamins. My four year old daughter adores dried mango pieces in her lunch box. Dried mango and apricots are rich in beta-carotene and iron. The downside, though, is that they tend to stick to the teeth, like sweets, so encourage children to brush their teeth afterwards, or follow with an apple or piece of cheese (this reduces the acidity and helps re-mineralise the tooth enamel).

Try packing carrot, pepper, celery or cucumber sticks (wrapped in clingfilm or in a small plastic pot) or putting salad vegetables (e.g. cherry tomatoes, tomatoes, cucumber) in sandwiches.

BEST FRUIT CHOICES	BEST VEGETABLE CHOICES
Apples, pears	Sticks of carrots, cucumber, peppers
Satsumas, clementines, mandarins	Baby sweetcorn
Bananas	Tomato, cucumber, lettuce or cress
Grapes	in a sandwich filling
Kiwi fruit (children can cut them in half and scoop out the flesh with a spoon)	Cherry tomatoes
Cherries	
Small container of strawberries, blueberries or raspberries	
Peaches, nectarines	
Small boxes of raisins	
Small bags of apricots, mango, pineapple, raisins, dried fruit mixtures	
Ring-pull cans or long-life cartons of fruit in juice	
Cartons and pots of fruit purée	

SANDWICHES AND FILLERS

Starchy carbohydrates should supply at least half of the calories in the lunchbox. This translates to about two slices of bread, or one large roll, or a small tub of pasta or rice. Sandwiches and rolls are a popular and easy choice. Vary their usual sandwiches by providing different types of bread. Try mini pitta bread pockets, tortilla wraps (cut into short lengths), a bagel or English muffins. Try making sandwiches with different types of bread, such as walnut bread, raisin or fruit bread, seeded bread or cheese and herb bread.

The filling should include a protein-rich food (such as cheese, chicken, ham, turkey, peanut butter, tuna or hummus) and, ideally, a salad vegetable (such as cucumber or tomato). Don't give jam, honey or chocolate-spread fillings too often as they contain mostly sugar and no protein. Save them as treats and instead provide some extra cheese or yoghurt.

Fed up with sandwiches? Pasta and rice salads can be jazzed up with chopped vegetables, nuts, dried fruit, beans, chopped chicken or tuna (see recipes pages 135, 139, 149).

The box below gives ideas for different sandwiches and healthy sandwich fillings.

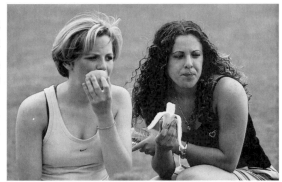

DAIRY PRODUCTS

Include one dairy food in the lunchbox (see the box below). Soya alternatives (e.g. soya 'cheese', soya 'yoghurt', soya milk and milkshakes) are also available if your children cannot tolerate dairy products. Both dairy and soya products supply protein as well as valuable calcium. Do check the label of yoghurts and fromage frais for artificial sweeteners, colours, and flavourings and try to keep these to a minimum. In general organic varieties and 'toddler' varieties are best as they don't contain additives. Yoghurt pouches and tubes of fromage frais are great for eating on the go as they don't require a spoon.

TREATS

Treats such as chocolate-coated bars, crisps and biscuits should not be included every day! They are loaded with fat and sugar and provide very little nutritional value.

BREADS/GRAINS	SANDWICH FILLINGS
Wholemeal, malted grain or wheatgerm bread	Lean ham and tomato
Wholemeal rolls	Peanut butter with grated cheese
Mini-pitta bread	Peanut butter with cucumber
English muffin	Marmite and cheese
Mini-bagel	Low fat soft cheese with tuna
Tortilla wrap	Mozzarella and tomato
Bread sticks	Hardboiled egg mixed with mayonnaise and cress
Wholemeal crackers	Banana and honey
Pot of potato salad	Turkey slices with cranberry sauce
Pot of pasta or rice salad	Avocado slices and chicken
	Hummus and grated carrot
	Cottage cheese and pineapple
	Salmon and cucumber
	Chopped chicken and coleslaw

These foods tend to cling to the teeth (yes, even savoury snacks), so unless children brush their teeth after lunch, these snacks can increase the chances of tooth decay.

A weekly treat is fine but encourage children to brush their teeth or eat a small piece of cheese afterwards — this helps counteract some of the damaging effects of sugar. My six year old daughter takes a fun travel toothbrush in her lunchbox, much to the initial amusement of her friends, who now join in the tooth brushing routine too!

A lot of parents provide a treat as a way of saying 'I'm thinking about you and I care for you'. But you can say this in other ways. Why not pop in a little note that says I love you, or a favourite cartoon, picture or joke? My daughter eagerly anticipates the surprise note or joke I put in her lunchbox, passes it around her friends and then collects the jokes in her special folder. At least she has a lasting reminder of lunchbox treats that don't damage her teeth!

LUNCHBOX DAIRY PRODUCTS

- Cheese in the sandwich filling
- Cheese portion
- Novelty cheese product (e.g. individual Cheddar portions, cheese strips or cheese strings)
- Carton or pouch of yoghurt
- Carton, pouch or tube of fromage frais
- Milk
- Milkshake
- Yoghurt drink
- Carton of custard

The box below gives ideas for healthier treats:

HEALTHY TREATS

- Scone
- Fruit bun or teacake
- Mini-pancake
- Cereal or breakfast bar
- Breadsticks
- Rice cakes
- Plain popcorn
- Plain reduced-fat crisps

- Homemade cakes and muffins (see recipes pages 170–175)
- Small bags of dried fruit (e.g. raisins, mango, apricots, dates, pineapple)

TWELVE LUNCHBOX IDEAS

1. Wholemeal chicken and tomato sandwich, a carton of yoghurt, carrot sticks, a satsuma and a drink of orange juice (diluted).

2. Peanut butter and cucumber roll, a cheese portion, strawberries, fromage frais and a bottle of water.

3. Slice of homemade pizza, strips of peppers, cherry tomatoes, an apple, yoghurt drink and a bottle of water.

4. Pasta salad with tuna, peppers and mushrooms, carton of yoghurt, small bag of dried apricots and an apple juice (diluted).

5. Tortilla wrap filled with cooked turkey and coleslaw, a small ring-pull tin of fruit in juice and a carton of milk.

6. Mini-bagel filled with soft cheese and sliced banana, a small bunch of grapes, a carton of fromage frais and a bottle of water.

7. Rice salad with cooked chicken, peas and sweetcorn, a pear, a carton of milkshake and a bottle of water.

8. Cooked tofu sausage or quorn sausage, wholemeal Marmite sandwich, small pot of nuts (e.g. cashews or peanuts), clementines, fruit juice (diluted).

9. Wholemeal crackers, hummus dip, cheese portion, grapes, a carton of yoghurt and a bottle of water.

10. Mini-pitta filled with tinned salmon and salad, cherries, mini box of raisins, a yoghurt drink and a bottle of water.

11. Wholemeal peanut butter sandwich, tub of mixed bean salad, a peach, a carton of custard and an orange juice (diluted).

12. Wholemeal roll filled with tuna, sweetcorn and mayonnaise, carrot sticks, cheese portion, small bag of dried fruit (e.g. mango, pineapple) and a bottle of water.

What's in school meals?

All school meals contracts should include nutritional standards for menu planning. Most use the guidelines prepared by the Caroline Walker Trust, which give the recommended nutrient content of an average school meal over a week. These guidelines are outlined in the box below.

Healthy eating at school

The National Healthy Schools Standards includes a healthy eating theme. The aim is to help schools become healthier by supporting the development and improvement of healthy school activities. These include providing healthier food at lunch and break times, and teaching children about healthy eating in the classroom.

NUTRITIONAL GUIDELINES FOR SCHOOL MEALS

Averaged over a period of a week, the school meal should provide:

- 30% of a child's calorie needs
- No more than 35% of a child's calories from fat
- No more than 11% of a child's calories from saturated fat
- At least 50% of a child's calories from carbohydrate
- No more than 11% of a child's calories from sugar
- At least 30% of a child's daily fibre needs
- At least 30% of a child's daily protein needs
- At least 30–40% of a child's iron, calcium, vitamin A, folate and vitamin C needs

What should I encourage children to eat for school lunch?

Some schools operate healthy eating initiatives, such as colour-coded healthy eating guides at lunch times. Here are a few guidelines:

	HEALTHIER OPTIONS	AVOID
Main course	Chicken or fish dishes (but not fried) Baked beans or bean hotpots Vegetable/chicken or lentil soup Pizza Pasta dishes with tomato or vegetable-based sauces Chicken, turkey or vegetable curries Jacket potatoes filled with tuna, baked beans, cheese or coleslaw Vegetable bakes and hotpots	Burgers Sausages Chicken nuggets Pies Fish in batter Pasta dishes with creamy or oily sauces Anything that appears excessively oily e.g. chilli, Bolognese sauce
Accompaniments	Potatoes — boiled, mashed or jacket	Chips Roast potatoes
Vegetables	At least one portion of vegetables or salad	
Dessert	Fresh fruit (at least three times a week) Fruit-based puddings, e.g. fruit crumble, banana custard Yoghurt Milk-based pudding, e.g. rice pudding	Cookies Cakes Sponge puddings Roly poly/suet pudding
Drinks	Water Fruit juice Milk	Fizzy drinks Fruit drinks, squash and soft drinks Sugar-free and 'diet' drinks

What can I give children after school?

Children always seem to be starving when they come home from school! Now is a good time to offer a healthy snack. It will bridge the gap between lunch and tea and, if they are playing sport or playing games, it will fuel their muscles and help their performance (see Chapter 7, 'Food for action').

Bread, toast, crackers and fruit are good choices as they are high in carbohydrate and also provide a range of vitamins and minerals. Balance the snack with a glass of milk, a handful of nuts or seeds, a carton of yoghurt or a piece of cheese. These foods all provide protein and calcium and, combined with a carbohydrate food, give a more sustained release of energy.

Don't give in to demands for sweets, biscuits and chocolate bars. It's easy to think that they 'deserve' a treat after school but, once they get into the healthy habit, they will be equally happy with healthy foods. My children and their friends delight in a plate of crackers, cheese and apple slices. Remember, sweets and biscuits provide only 'empty calories' and will not give lasting energy. They are high GI foods (see page 29), giving a rapid rise in blood sugar, followed by a rapid fall. The result? Flagging energy levels, poor concentration and hunger. If they will be playing sport, they will need a snack that will help keep up their energy and stop them tiring before the end. Even if they will be doing homework or a similar sedentary activity, they will need a snack that will maintain concentration and stave off hunger.

The box on the next page gives some ideas for after-school snacks.

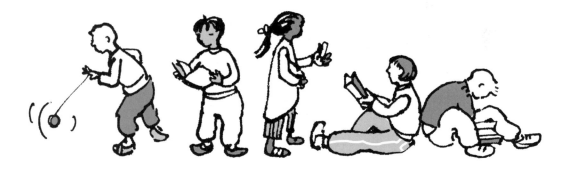

AFTER-SCHOOL SNACKS

Accompany with a drink of water or diluted fruit juice (one part juice to one part water)

- A piece of fresh fruit and a glass of milk
- Wholemeal toast and Marmite with a handful of nuts
- Cereal bar, breakfast bar or energy bar
- A carton of yoghurt and a small bag of dried fruit
- A bowl of breakfast cereal with milk
- Mini-pancake or scone and a carton of fromage frais
- Crackers with cheese
- Homemade fruit muffins or cakes (see recipes pages 170–175)
- Fruit smoothies
- Peanut butter sandwich

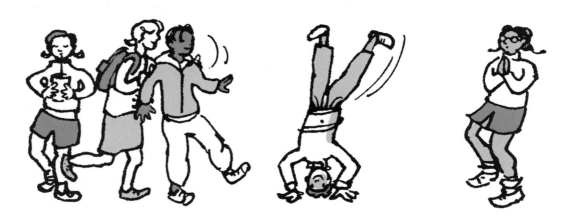

12 EATING DISORDERS

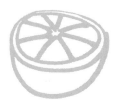

It is not unusual for young teenagers to become more body-conscious, but when they become preoccupied with their weight, and develop negative thoughts about their appearance this could signal the beginning of an eating disorder. Eating disorders are increasingly common among children and teenagers, especially girls. Surveys have revealed that an alarming number of normal weight girls perceive themselves as overweight and want to lose weight. Ninety per cent of children and teenagers with eating disorders are girls.

This chapter will help you to decide whether the teenager you know may have an eating disorder. It describes the warning signs and offers some explanation as to why some young girls, and athletes in particular, develop eating disorders. It gives some suggestions for supporting children with eating disorders, and how to prevent them.

What are eating disorders?

Generally, eating disorders involve negative, self-critical thoughts and feelings about appearance and food. Sufferers are preoccupied about food and their weight. Food may be seen as a penalty for perceived failure or as a source of comfort. By controlling their food intake, sufferers believe that they are in control of one particular situation. A person with anorexia literally starves themselves thin, eating very little or no food. Bulimia is a condition of bingeing and purging, where a person secretly eats vast quantities of food and then regurgitates it either orally by making themselves sick, or by misusing laxatives.

- In a survey of 12–14 year old girls, 12% admitted to binge-eating, and 7% said they used self-induced vomiting to lose weight (Source: Princess Margaret Hospital, Toronto).

- Eating disorder clinics report that girls as young as eight are being admitted for the treatment of eating disorders.

- Many 5 year old girls are already concerned with their shape and about being fat (Source: Women's Hospital, Boston).

- 70% of normal weight girls aged 11–18 years thought they were too fat (Source: Institute of Psychiatry).

- Up to 62% of girls involved in certain sports such as gymnastics and endurance running have abnormal eating behaviour.

What are the causes of eating disorders?

There is no single cause, rather a whole series of circumstances or pressures that make a person develop an eating disorder. It may be triggered by a life event, such as a divorce, illness or death in the family, or, for others, an insignificant event, such as a comment made about their weight. But there are nearly always other underlying factors involved. These can include family problems, relationships, a low self-esteem, problems at school, and a fear of failure. There may also be an intense desire for athletic success at sport and a belief that weight loss will allow them to perform better in competition.

It is worth remembering that adolescence is a difficult time for young girls, as they need to adjust to their changing body shape as well as the responsibilities of growing up. They also need to deal with pressures of exams and other adolescent stresses, such as their developing sexuality and their identity as young women.

Why are eating disorders common among young athletes?

Eating disorders are more common among teenagers involved in sports where a low body weight or body fat percentage is thought to be advantageous: endurance running, figure skating, gymnastics and dancing. In susceptible girls, the demands of certain sports or the requests made by coaches to lose weight may trigger an eating disorder. For example, in their determination to improve their performance and achieve competitive success, some girls mistakenly believe that thinness will lead to greater success in their sport. They then become obsessed with weight loss. They may identify with elite athletes in their particular sport who are inherently slim — natural ectomorphs (see Chapter 9, page 81) — and model themselves on their thin physiques. Of course, there are many other factors to achieving success,

PARENTS AND FOOD

Do you have a healthy attitude to food? Do you worry about your own weight and shape? Have you regularly dieted or tried to watch your weight? Some experts believe that children's attitudes to food and their body image may be passed down from their parents. Children learn by example. If children see their mothers shunning snack foods or counting calories they are likely to do the same. A mother's neurosis about food may rub off on her daughter.

1. A study involving 100 young children concluded that dieting parents or those who are over-anxious about food, may be to blame for their children's unhealthy attitude towards eating and their bodies (Source: Glasgow University).

2. Mothers who dislike body fat are communicating that attitude to their children (Source: St Mary's Hospital, London).

3. Over-protective, uncommunicative parents are more likely to raise children who will develop an eating disorder (Source: Manchester University).

including training, natural ability and mental preparation. Nutrition is essential for training, so if athletes cut down on their calorie intake their performance will suffer. Misguided weight loss attempts are counterproductive as they produce instead a negative effect on an athlete's performance.

Girls with a personality predisposed to eating disorders may be attracted to certain sports, such as endurance running because they see it as another method of weight loss. They may compete at events, but their main motivation to run remains the pursuit of slimness.

How do I know if an athlete has an eating disorder?

Look at the lists of warning signs for anorexia nervosa and bulimia nervosa in the box below. These will help you to recognise potential problems in your teenage athletes. The presence of only one or two signs does not necessarily mean that they

WARNING SIGNS FOR ANOREXIA NERVOSA	WARNING SIGNS FOR BULIMIA NERVOSA
• Dramatic loss of weight	• Extreme weight fluctuations
• Preoccupation with food, calories and weight	• Swollen salivary glands
• Exercising excessively	• Irregular periods
• Mood swings	• Excessive concern about weight
• Avoiding social situations where food is served	• Visits bathroom during or after meals
• Periods stop or have never started	• Increasingly self-critical of her body and performance
• Feeling fat even when underweight	• Emotional and depressed, mood swings
• Setting unreasonably high standards	• Feel out of control
• Lying about eating meals and refuses to eat in company	• Eat large amounts of food followed by strict dieting
	• Takes laxatives or diuretics

have an eating disorder. *It is important to seek advice from an appropriate health professional for a proper diagnosis and the right kind of help.*

How will an eating disorder affect their health and performance?

Eating too little over a period of time can be physically and emotionally harmful. Initially, anorexic athletes appear to have endless energy and are capable of pushing themselves through hard training sessions. But as sufferers lose more weight, their athletic performance drops. They will eventually feel too tired to train as their bodies become too weak. Rather than helping them perform better in sport, eating too little will ultimately cause them to stop exercising altogether.

In girls, menstruation usually stops (or doesn't start in young teens), increasing the risk of brittle bones. They may suffer repeated injuries and stress fractures and, in the long term, risk premature osteoporosis.

Many athletes with bulimia appear to cope with training but inside they feel out of control and worthless. Repeated use of laxatives, diuretics and making themselves sick can damage their health. They can develop bad breath, dental erosion and decay, dehydration, kidney and bowel problems.

What can I do if I think a child has an eating disorder?

If you suspect a child may be worrying too much about their weight or developing an eating disorder there are a number of things you can do to help. Talk to them and listen to their concerns, but avoid making comments about their appearance. Whatever you say about their appearance may be misinterpreted. Instead, show lots of love and respect. If they deny that they have a problem, keep persevering. Sufferers do their best to keep it a secret as long as possible, but often they want help and do not know whom to ask. They may feel embarrassed and their self-esteem threatened, so you must avoid a direct confrontation about their weight loss or eating behaviour. Do not present them with 'evidence' of their disorder. Instead, let them know that you are there if they need to talk and offer unconditional support. Don't fight with them about food.

Once they have admitted to having a problem, encourage them to seek help. You can listen, but don't try to give advice if you are not qualified to do so. The earlier a problem is identified the shorter the treatment period and the better the chances of treatment. There are various places that you can go to for help, including trained counsellors from a self-help organisation (see Resources) or to a GP who will be able to refer them to psychologists and dietitians specialising in eating disorders.

Preventing eating disorders

Your own behaviour may help children avoid eating disorders. Focus on their strengths and you will build self-esteem. Here are some pointers to foster a positive body image and prevent eating disorders:

- Support your children for what they are as well as what they do or what they look like.
- Be a healthy example — avoid making negative comments about your own body (e.g. 'I'm fat') in front of children and teenagers.
- Aim for moderation in food and exercise — your children will be more likely to do as you do.
- Teach children to feel good about themselves, regardless of body size or shape.
- Reassure adolescents that the physical changes they are experiencing are normal, and that everyone develops at their own rate.
- Discuss body image issues as they arise — always give reassurance and emphasise your child's individuality.
- Help your children develop a critical awareness of the images and messages portrayed in the media.
- Never use food as a punishment or reward.
- Emphasise nutrition and enjoyment — look at the health-giving properties of food rather than the calories or fat.
- Do not force your children to eat when they are not hungry — encourage them to listen to their natural appetite cues.
- Do not pressurise your children to eat only low fat healthy food or

ban fatty foods or sweets — this could have the opposite effect to that intended.

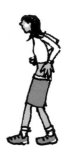

- Mealtimes should not be stressful.
- Encourage children to enjoy all forms of physical activities and to appreciate that movement is fun. Exercise should not be portrayed as a method of weight loss.
- Parents who follow a weight loss diet should emphasise that this is not right for a child.

13 KIDS' MENU PLANS

Use the following menu plans to help you feed your children the right balance of carbohydrate, protein, fat, vitamins and minerals. Remember, the emphasis should be on variety and enjoyment. Introduce new foods and flavours at every opportunity. Make healthy snacks easily accessible and limit the amount of unhealthy food in your household. Encourage your children to drink 6–8 glasses of fluid (water, diluted fruit juice, milk) daily and an additional 350–700 ml for each hour of exercise (see Chapter 8, 'Drinking for action').

There are two seven day menu plans for 5–10 year olds and two seven day menu plans for 11–15 year olds, each including a vegetarian eating plan. Judge the portion sizes according to your children's age, appetite and specific requirements (see Chapter 2, 'What should active children eat?').

SEVEN DAY MENU PLAN FOR **5–10 YEAR OLDS**

MONDAY	Breakfast	Wholegrain cereal with milk Banana
	Lunchbox	Tuna, cucumber and mayonnaise wholemeal sandwich Small ring-pull can of fruit in juice Carton of yoghurt Water
	Supper	Chicken Burgers (see recipe page 156) Oven Potato Wedges (see recipe page 162) Baked beans, broccoli Stewed apples and raisins
TUESDAY	Breakfast	Wholemeal toast and peanut butter or Marmite Fresh fruit Milk or yoghurt
	Lunchbox	Slice of pizza Carrot and cucumber crudités A bunch of seedless grapes Carton of fromage frais Orange juice
	Supper	Pasta and Tuna Bake (see recipe page 136) Sliced tomatoes with a little dressing Yoghurt and fruit pudding
WEDNESDAY	Breakfast	Porridge made with milk and water A little honey and raisins
	Lunchbox	Pitta bread filled with cold chopped chicken and coleslaw Dried apricots Milk
	Supper	Toad-and-Vegetables-in-the-Hole (see recipe page 135) Spring cabbage or broccoli Fresh fruit
THURSDAY	Breakfast	Banana Smoothie (see recipe page 176)
	Lunchbox	Wholemeal roll filled with lean ham and tomato Piece of fresh fruit Carton of custard, water

	Supper	Jacket potato filled with baked beans and grated cheese OR filled with scrambled egg and tomato Crunchy Apple Crumble (see recipe page 165)
FRIDAY	Breakfast	Bowl of fresh fruit, e.g. oranges, pineapple and mango Carton of fruit yoghurt
	Lunchbox	Cheese dip or Hummus (see recipe page 167), breadsticks Crudités, e.g. carrot, pepper and cucumber strips Small box of raisins Milkshake
	Supper	Chicken Baked in Tomato Sauce (see recipe page 131) Boiled rice, peas Fresh fruit
SATURDAY	Breakfast	Boiled egg and wholemeal toast Orange juice
	Lunch	Potato soup (see recipe page 151) Grated cheese Granary roll Fresh fruit salad (see recipes pages 167–168)
	Supper	Homemade Chicken Nuggets (see recipe page 155) Mighty Root Mash (see recipe page 161) Carrots and peas Baked Rice Pudding (see recipe page 165)
SUNDAY	Breakfast	Pancakes Filled with Apple Purée (see recipe page 164)
	Lunch	Jacket potato Grilled chicken Broccoli and carrots Raspberry Fool (see recipe page 163)
	Supper	Cheese and Tomato Pizza (see recipe page 160) with any of the suggested toppings Salad: cherry tomatoes, peppers, grated carrot, cucumber A little salad dressing Fresh fruit

SEVEN DAY MENU PLAN FOR   **10–15 YEAR OLDS**

MONDAY	Breakfast	Porridge made with milk and water Raisins
	Lunchbox	Bagel with low-fat soft cheese and tinned salmon or tuna Cherry tomatoes Carton of yoghurt A piece of fresh fruit Bottle of water
	Supper	Vegetable and Pasta Soup (see recipe page 154) Wholemeal roll Banana and Nut Fool (see recipe page 167)
TUESDAY	Breakfast	English muffin or bagel with jam or honey Yoghurt or milk
	Lunchbox	Small container of pasta salad with tuna Satsuma or kiwi fruit Small bag or pot of nuts and raisins Fruit juice
	Supper	Fish Pie (see recipe page 133) Broccoli and carrots Baked Bananas (see recipe page 166)
WEDNESDAY	Breakfast	Wholegrain cereal with milk Fresh fruit Wholemeal toast and honey
	Lunchbox	Wholemeal roll with turkey and cranberry sauce Crudités, e.g. cucumber, pepper and carrot strips Cheese portion Piece of fresh fruit Bottle of water
	Supper	Pasta with Sweetcorn and Tuna (see recipe page 135) Brussels sprouts or broccoli Poached pears

THURSDAY	Breakfast	Mango and Strawberry Smoothie (see recipe page 177)
	Lunchbox	Thermos of tomato or vegetable soup Wholemeal roll with cheese Small bag of dried apricots Bottle of water
	Supper	Grilled chicken Jacket potato Baby sweetcorn and sugar snap peas
FRIDAY	Breakfast	Muesli with milk or yoghurt Strawberries or raspberries
	Lunchbox	Wholemeal egg and mayonnaise sandwich Cucumber slices Carton of yoghurt Banana Muffin (see recipe page 171) Bottle of water
	Supper	Fish Cakes (see recipe page 139) Carrots and peas Banana Bread Pudding (see recipe page 166)
SATURDAY	Breakfast	Pancakes Filled with Fresh Fruit (see recipe page 164)
	Lunch	Butternut Squash Soup (see recipe page 153) Wholemeal roll Fresh fruit salad with frozen yoghurt
	Supper	Pasta Turkey Bolognese (see recipe page 132) Broccoli and cauliflower Crunchy Apple Crumble (see recipe page 165)
SUNDAY	Breakfast	Boiled egg and wholemeal toast Nectarine or a pear
	Lunch	Golden Baked Chicken (see recipe page 133) Mashed potatoes and green beans Fresh fruit salad with frozen yoghurt or custard
	Supper	Sardines on wholemeal toast Baked beans and coleslaw Yoghurt and Fruit Pudding (see recipe page 166)

SEVEN DAY VEGETARIAN MENU PLAN FOR **5–10 YEAR OLDS**

MONDAY	Breakfast	Muesli with milk or yoghurt Orange juice
	Lunchbox	Spicy Bean Burger (see recipe page 156) wrapped in foil Small wholemeal roll Crudités, e.g. carrots, peppers, cucumber A piece of fruit Carton of yoghurt Bottle of water
	Supper	Vegetarian Spaghetti Bolognese (see recipe page 140) Fresh fruit with custard or frozen yoghurt
TUESDAY	Breakfast	Porridge made with milk, water, honey Raisins
	Lunchbox	Wholemeal peanut butter and cucumber sandwich Small bag of dried apricots Novelty cheese portion Orange juice
	Supper	Broccoli and Cheese Soup (see recipe page 152) Wholemeal roll Baked Bananas with yoghurt (see recipe page 166)
WEDNESDAY	Breakfast	Banana Milkshake (see recipe page 176) Wholemeal toast and Marmite
	Lunchbox	Mini-bagel filled with soft cheese and banana Satsuma Carton of custard Orange juice
	Supper	Potato and Cheese Pie (see recipe page 147) Green beans and carrots Baked Rice Pudding with fresh fruit (see recipe page 165)
THURSDAY	Breakfast	Wholegrain cereal with milk Orange juice
	Lunchbox	Hummus dip (see recipe page 169) Breadsticks or crackers Crudités, e.g. carrot, pepper and cucumber strips Small pot of fruit purée Carton of fromage frais Bottle of water

	Supper	Spicy Lentil Burgers (see recipe page 157) Jacket potato Baked beans and broccoli Fresh fruit salad
FRIDAY	Breakfast	Wholemeal toast and jam or marmalade Fresh fruit e.g. apple or strawberries Milk or yoghurt
	Lunchbox	Mini-pitta with grated cheese and tomato Small pot of nuts, e.g. almonds, cashews, peanuts Piece of fresh fruit Apple Muffin (see recipe page 170) Bottle of water
	Supper	Marvellous Macaroni Cheese (see recipe page 141) Cauliflower and broccoli Raspberry Fool (see recipe page 163)
SATURDAY	Breakfast	Poached egg Tomatoes Wholemeal toast with Marmite
	Lunch	Carrot Soup (see recipe page 153) with grated cheese Wholemeal roll Baked apple stuffed with raisins, chopped dates, almonds and honey
	Supper	Butter Bean and Leek Supper (see recipe page 145) New potatoes and carrots Yoghurt
SUNDAY	Breakfast	Pancakes Filled with Fresh Fruit (see recipe page 164) Orange juice
	Lunch	Nut Burgers (see recipe page 158) Jacket potato Carrots and Brussels sprouts or broccoli Banana Bread Pudding (see recipe page 166)
	Supper	Cheese on wholemeal toast Tomatoes and cucumber Yoghurt

SEVEN DAY VEGETARIAN MENU PLAN FOR   10–15 YEAR OLDS

MONDAY	Breakfast	English muffin or bagel with a slice of cheese Fresh fruit
	Lunchbox	Pot of pasta salad with red kidney beans, peppers and tomatoes Carton of yoghurt Small bag of dried fruit Bottle of water
	Supper	Cauliflower cheese Jacket potato and green beans Baked Bananas (see recipe page 166)
TUESDAY	Breakfast	Wholegrain cereal with milk Raisins or dried apricots
	Lunchbox	Wholemeal roll with sliced avocado and tomato Cheese portion Piece of fresh fruit Carton of milkshake
	Supper	Cheese and Tomato Pizza (see recipe page 159) with any of the suggested toppings Jacket potato Coleslaw Fresh fruit
WEDNESDAY	Breakfast	Porridge made with milk and water Banana
	Lunchbox	Thermos of vegetable soup Wholemeal roll Small bunch of seedless grapes Orange juice
	Supper	Chickpea and Spinach Pasta (see recipe page 142) Fresh fruit salad with yoghurt or custard
THURSDAY	Breakfast	Muesli mixed with grated apple Milk or yoghurt
	Lunchbox	Cooked vegetarian sausage, wrapped in foil Wholemeal Marmite sandwich Small pot of nuts (e.g. almonds, cashews, peanuts) Carton of fromage frais Bottle of water

	Supper	Bean Burritos (see recipe page 144) Salad or broccoli Stewed pears with raisins and honey
FRIDAY	Breakfast	Energiser (see recipe page 177) Wholemeal toast
	Lunchbox	English muffin with peanut butter and cheese Carrot sticks Carton of yoghurt Small bag of dried fruit Fruit juice
	Supper	Vegetable Korma (see recipe page 146) Rice Fresh fruit salad
SATURDAY	Breakfast	Scrambled egg with mushrooms Wholemeal toast
	Lunch	Spicy Bean Burger (see recipe page 156) Wholemeal bap Salad Fresh fruit
	Supper	Jacket potato filled with stir-fried vegetables or ratatouille Crunchy apple crumble (or other fruit variety) (see recipe page 165) Custard or yoghurt
SUNDAY	Breakfast	Pancakes Filled with Sliced Bananas and Honey (see recipe page 164)
	Lunch	Red Lentil Dahl Rice Carrots and broccoli Cherry Clafouti (see recipe page 167)
	Supper	Real Tomato Soup (see recipe page 152) with grated cheese Wholemeal roll Fresh fruit

AFTER-SCHOOL SNACKS AND LUNCHBOX TREATS

Wholemeal chicken, tuna or cheese sandwich

Wholemeal banana or honey sandwich

Wholemeal toast with Marmite or peanut butter

Crackers, oatcakes or rice cakes with a little cheese

Yoghurt drink

Individual cheese portion

Nuts — peanuts, cashews, almonds

Sesame snaps

Crudités, e.g. carrots, peppers, cucumbers and celery

Hummus (see recipe page 169)

Fresh fruit, e.g. apple slices, pear, clementines, grapes, strawberries

Carton of yoghurt and fresh fruit

Dried fruit (e.g. raisins, apricots, apple rings, mango) and cheese

Mini-pancake or scone

Wholegrain breakfast cereal with milk

Plain popcorn

Apple Muffins (see recipe page 170)

Fruit Muffins (see recipe page 170)

Banana Muffins (see recipe page 171)

Apple Spice Cake (see recipe page 172)

Carrot Cake (see recipe page 172)

Fruit Cake (see recipe page 173)

Ginger Spice Cake (see recipe page 173)

Wholemeal Raisin Biscuits (see recipe page 174)

Apricot Bar (see recipe page 174)

Milkshake, e.g. Strawberry and Banana Milkshake (see recipe page 178)

Smoothie, e.g. Banana Smoothie (see recipe page 176)

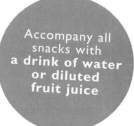

Accompany all snacks with **a drink of water or diluted fruit juice**

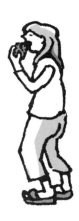

AFTER-SPORT SNACKS

Bananas

Fresh fruit — grapes, apples, satsumas, pears

Dried fruit — raisins, apricots, dates

Fruit bar or liquorice bar

Crackers and rice cakes with bananas or cheese

Roll, sandwich, English muffin or bagel with honey, jam or Marmite

Cereal or muesli bar

Energy bar

Fruit yoghurt

Milkshake (see recipes pages 176–178)

Smoothie (see recipes pages 176–178)

Home-made Cereal Bar (see recipe page 175)

Banana Muffins (see recipe page 171)

Banana Loaf (see recipe page 171)

Wholemeal Raisin Biscuits (see recipe page 174)

Accompany all snacks with a drink of water, diluted fruit juice or isotonic sports drink

MAIN MEALS

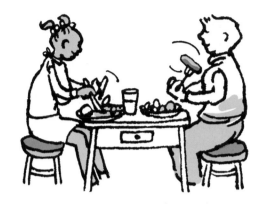

CHICKEN BAKED IN TOMATO SAUCE

Anything in tomato sauce will be a hit with most children so you can use this as a good opportunity to disguise extra vegetables.

Makes 4 servings

To balance the meal, add jacket potato and carrots

4 chicken portions, on the bone
2 tbsp (30 ml) olive oil
I onion, chopped
2 garlic cloves, crushed
I red and I green pepper, chopped
I tin (400 g) chopped tomatoes
I tbsp (I5 ml) each of fresh basil, fresh parsley and fresh chives (alternatively, use I tbsp (I5 ml) dried mixed herbs)

I Pre-heat the oven to 160°C/ 325°F/ gas mark 3.

2 Sauté the chicken portions in I tablespoon of the olive oil until browned. Remove with a slotted spoon and put in a casserole dish.

3 Heat the remaining oil. Add the onion and garlic and cook for 3 minutes.

4 Add the peppers and cook for a further 2 minutes. Add the tinned tomatoes and herbs and simmer for 5 minutes.

5 Spoon sauce over the chicken and cook in the oven for about 45 minutes.

CHICKEN CURRY

Make this dish more nutritious by adding extra vegetables to the curry sauce. Adjust the amount of curry paste according to your children's taste.

Makes 4 servings

1 tbsp (15 ml) olive oil
2 chicken breasts, boneless, skinned and cut into strips
1 onion, chopped
1 clove of garlic, crushed
2 tbsp (30 ml) mild curry paste
1 tin (400 g) chopped tomatoes
125 g (4 oz) cauliflower florets
125 g (4 oz) carrots, sliced
125 g (4 oz) frozen peas
60g (2oz) sultanas

To balance the meal, add basmati rice or mini naan breads.

1 Heat the olive oil in a large heavy bottomed pan and cook the chicken strips for 5 minutes until brown. Put aside on a plate.
2 Add the onion and sauté for 5 minutes.
3 Add the curry paste, tinned tomatoes and vegetables, stir then bring to the boil. Simmer for 10 minutes.
4 Return the chicken to the pan with the sultanas, and continue cooking for a further 10 minutes.

PASTA TURKEY BOLOGNESE

Turkey mince is used in place of the conventional beef. It is high in protein and low in fat. Bolognese sauce is a good way of hiding vegetables and beans.

Makes 4 servings

1 tbsp (15 ml) olive oil
300 g (10 oz) turkey mince
1 large onion, chopped
2 sticks of celery
2 carrots, grated
1 tin (400 g) chopped tomatoes
1 tin (420 g) red kidney beans
1 teaspoon (5 ml) dried mixed herbs
Salt and freshly ground black pepper
175 g (6 oz) spaghetti or other pasta shapes (adjust the quantity according to your children's appetite)

To balance the meal, add broccoli or spring cabbage.

1 Heat the olive oil in a large pan and sauté the turkey mince until it is browned. Add the onions and cook for a further 3–4 minutes.
2 Add the celery and carrots and cook for a further 5 minutes until just tender.
3 Stir in the chopped tomatoes, red kidney beans and herbs. Bring to the boil and simmer for 5 minutes. Season with salt and black pepper.
4 Meanwhile, cook the pasta according to the directions on the packet. Drain, then stir into the Bolognese sauce.

GOLDEN BAKED CHICKEN

This is one of the easiest and healthiest ways to cook chicken and proves that you don't need a packet mix to tempt children to eat their food.

Makes 4 servings

4 chicken breasts, boneless and skinless
60 g (2 oz) flour
1 tbsp (15 ml) paprika
2 tbsp (30 ml) olive oil
Salt and freshly ground black pepper to taste

To balance the meal, add green beans and mashed potatoes.

1 Pre-heat the oven to 180°C/ 350°F/ gas mark 4.

2 Place flour and paprika in a plastic bag. Add the chicken breasts and shake until the chicken is well coated.

3 Put the olive oil in a baking dish. Add the chicken breasts and turn carefully in the oil. Cover with foil and bake for 20 minutes.

4 Remove the foil and bake for a further 10 minutes until the chicken is golden brown.

FISH PIE

This popular children's meal is made healthier by adding swede to the mashed potato. You can substitute parsnips or squash if you prefer.

Makes 4 servings

300 g (10 oz) potatoes, peeled and cut into large chunks
300 g (10 oz) swede, peeled and cut into large chunks
550 g (1¼ lb) cod fillets
600ml (1 pint) skimmed milk
1 bay leaf
25 g (1 oz) butter
2 large leeks, thinly sliced
2 heaped tbsp plain flour
Salt, freshly ground black pepper, 1 tsp (5 ml) Dijon mustard
60 g (2 oz) mature Cheddar cheese, grated

To balance the meal, add broccoli and peas.

1 Pre-heat the oven to 190°C/375°F/ gas mark 5.

2 Cook the potatoes and swede in fast-boiling water for about 15 minutes or until soft. Drain and mash with about one third of the milk.

3 Meanwhile place the cod in a saucepan with the remaining milk and bay leaf. Bring to the boil and simmer for about 5 minutes.

4 Strain the milk into a jug. Roughly flake the fish.

5 Melt the butter in a pan, add the leeks and cook for 5 minutes until softened. Stir in the flour. Slowly add the milk, stirring continuously over a low heat until the sauce has thickened. Season with salt, pepper and Dijon mustard.

6 Combine the sauce with the leeks and fish. Place in a baking dish.

7 Cover evenly with the mashed potatoes and swede and scatter the cheese on top.

8 Bake for 20 minutes until the top is golden brown.

LITTLE CHICKEN AND VEGETABLE PARCELS

These pies are made with filo pastry, which contains less fat than shortcrust pastry. You can substitute different vegetables for those suggested in the recipe — they will count towards the 5 daily servings of vegetables and fruit recommended for children.

Makes 8 small parcels

2 chicken breasts, skinless and boneless
2 tbsp (30 ml) olive oil
85 g (3 oz) button mushrooms, sliced
1 medium courgette, chopped
2 carrots, thinly sliced
2 tsp (10 ml) cornflour
200 ml (7 fl oz) milk
175 g (6 oz) filo pastry

To balance the meal, add Potato Wedges (Page 162) and a green vegetable.

1 Cut the chicken into small pieces. Heat 1 tbsp of the oil in a pan. Add the chicken and sauté over a high heat for 3 minutes.

2 Add the vegetables and continue cooking over a moderate heat for 5–6 minutes until the vegetables are softened.

3 Stir in the cornflour. Slowly add the milk, stirring continuously until the sauce has thickened. Remove from the heat.

4 Cut the pastry into 24 squares each measuring 13 cm × 13 cm (5 in × 5 in). Lightly brush one square with olive oil, cover with another square and brush with oil. Cover with a third square.

5 Place a spoonful of the filling in the centre of the square. Brush the edges with a little water. Fold over one corner of the pastry to make a triangle and press to seal. Repeat with the remaining pastry squares until you have 8 parcels.

6 Place the parcels on a lightly oiled baked tray and brush with olive oil. Bake in the oven for 15–20 minutes until golden brown.

TOAD-AND-VEGETABLES-IN-THE-HOLE

This variation of Toad-in-the-Hole includes tasty root vegetables, which add extra vitamins and fibre to the meal. It is a good dish to serve to vegetarians, too, as you can substitute vegetarian sausages for the meat ones.

Makes 4 servings

4 carrots
1 parsnip
225 g (8 oz) butternut squash
2 tbsp (30 ml) sunflower oil
4 lean beef sausages or vegetarian sausages
125 g (4 oz) plain flour
1 egg
300 ml (½ pint) milk

To balance the meal, add a green vegetable.

1 Pre-heat the oven to 190°C/ 375°F/ gas mark 5.

2 Cut the vegetables into 2½ cm (1 in) chunks. Place in a roasting tin, drizzle over the sunflower oil and toss to coat. Bake in the oven for 20 minutes.

3 Prick the sausages. Add to the roasting tin and cook in the oven for a further 10 minutes.

4 Meanwhile make the batter. Place the flour, egg and milk in a liquidiser and blend until smooth.

5 Spoon the roasted vegetables and sausages into a rectangular dish. Pour over the batter and bake for a further 40 minutes until the batter has risen and is crisp on the outside.

PASTA WITH SWEETCORN AND TUNA

This dish is quick to prepare and makes a good midweek standby. It's also good eaten cold as a lunchbox salad.

Makes 4 servings

175 g (6 oz) pasta shapes (adjust the quantity according to your children's appetite)
1 tbsp (15 ml) olive oil
1 onion, chopped
1 garlic clove, crushed
1 tin (400g) chopped tomatoes
1 tbsp (15 ml) tomato purée
125 g (4 oz) sweetcorn
1 tin (200g) tuna in water or brine, drained and flaked
1 tsp (5 ml) dried basil

To balance the meal, add broccoli or Brussels sprouts.

1 Cook the pasta according to the directions on the packet. Drain.

2 Meanwhile, place the onion, garlic and tomatoes in a large non-stick frying pan and cook for 4–5 minutes until onion is soft.

3 Stir in the tomato purée, chopped tomatoes and sweetcorn and cook for 5 minutes.

4 Add the tuna and basil and heat through.

5 Stir the Sweetcorn and Tuna sauce into the pasta and serve.

PASTA WITH HAM AND MUSHROOM SAUCE

Makes 4 servings

175 g (6 oz) pasta shells (adjust quantity depending on appetite)
1 tbsp (15 ml) olive oil
4 slices (125 g) ham (preferably reduced salt), chopped
125 g (4 oz) small mushrooms, halved
1 tbsp (15 ml) cornflour
300ml (½ pint) milk
1 tsp dried oregano
Freshly ground black pepper

To balance the meal, add carrots and a green vegetable.

1 Cook the pasta according to directions on the packet. Drain.

2 Meanwhile, heat the olive oil in a large frying pan. Cook the ham and mushrooms for 4–5 minutes.

3 Stir in the cornflour together with a little milk. Gradually add the rest of the milk, stirring continuously.

4 Heat until the sauce just reaches boiling point. Remove from the heat and stir in the herbs and pepper.

5 Combine with the cooked pasta.

PASTA AND TUNA BAKE

This recipe makes a balanced meal in itself. The tuna and milk provide protein, the pasta provides energy-giving carbohydrate and the vegetables provide vitamins and fibre.

Makes 4 servings

175 g (6 oz) pasta shells (adjust the quantity according to appetite)
1 tbsp (15 ml) olive oil
1 onion, sliced
2 sticks of celery, chopped
1 green pepper, chopped
125 g (4 oz) frozen peas
1 tbsp (15 ml) fresh parsley, chopped
1 tin (200g) tuna in water or brine

White Sauce:
1 tbsp (15 ml) butter
1 tbsp (15 ml) cornflour
300 ml (½ pint) milk

To balance the meal, add fresh fruit for dessert.

1 Preheat the oven to 180°C/ 375°F/ gas mark 5.

2 Cook the pasta. Drain.

3 In a non-stick frying pan, heat the olive oil. Sauté the onion for 3 min until translucent, then celery, pepper and peas. Continue cooking for a further 5 min.

4 White sauce: melt butter in a pan, stir in cornflour, then add the milk slowly, stirring over a low/medium heat until thickened.

5 Spread a thin layer of vegetables onto the bottom of a baking dish. Cover with a layer of pasta, then flaked tuna. Add a layer of white sauce. Sprinkle parsley between each layer. Repeat the process. Finish with white sauce on top.

6 Bake for 20 minutes.

LASAGNE

Choosing lean mince keeps the saturated fat content of this recipe to a minimum. Include other varieties of vegetables, such as mushrooms and spinach, instead of the celery and pepper, if you wish. This dish is a good way of hiding those vegetables!

Makes 4 servings

1 tbsp (15 ml) olive oil
1 onion, chopped
1 celery stick, chopped
1 red pepper, chopped
225 g (8 oz) lean beef mince (or turkey mince)
1 tin (400g) chopped tomatoes
2 tbsp (30 ml) tomato puree
1 tsp (5 ml) dried basil or oregano
Salt and freshly ground black pepper to taste
8 sheets lasagne (the no pre-cook variety)
85 g (3 oz) mozzarella cheese

To balance the meal, add fresh fruit for dessert.

1 Preheat the oven to 180°C/ 350°F/ gas mark 4.

2 Heat the olive oil in a large non-stick frying pan. Cook the onion, celery, pepper and mince, stirring frequently, for 5–6 minutes until the mince is browned. Drain off any fat.

3 Add the tomatoes, tomato puree, and herbs. Season with salt and pepper to taste.

4 Place a layer of lasagne sheets at the bottom of an oiled baking dish. Spoon over one third of the mince mixture. Repeat the layers, finishing with a layer of the mince mixture.

5 Cover with very thin slices of mozzarella. Bake for 30 minutes until the cheese is bubbling and golden.

CHILLI CON CARNE

This version of the classic dish smuggles in extra vegetables. You may use any type of lean minced meat such as turkey, beef or pork.

Makes 4 servings

225 g (8 oz) lean minced turkey, beef or pork
1 tbsp (15 ml) olive oil
1 onion, chopped
1 garlic clove, crushed
1 green pepper, chopped
1 celery stick, chopped
85 g (3 oz) button mushrooms, whole or cut in half
1 tsp (5 ml) paprika
1 pinch chilli powder (according to your children's tastes)
½ tsp (2.5 ml) ground cumin
2 tbsp (30 ml) tomato puree
400 ml (¾ pint) stock or water
1 tin (420g) red kidney beans

To balance the meal, add boiled rice and a green vegetable.

1 Dry-fry the mince in a non-stick pan for about 5 minutes until browned. Drain off any fat. Set aside.

2 Heat the olive oil in a large pan and sauté the onion, pepper, celery, mushrooms and garlic for about 3 minutes. Add the spices and fry for a further minute.

3 Add the tomato puree, stock or water, and the beans. Cover and simmer for about 1 hour.

CHICKEN AND MIXED PEPPER RISOTTO

Peppers are bursting with vitamin C and other antioxidants. This recipe is a great way of introducing them to children.

Makes 4 servings

1 tbsp (15 ml) olive oil
1 onion, chopped
1 red pepper, cut into thin strips
1 yellow pepper, cut into thin strips
175 g (6 oz) long-grain or Arborio rice
1 l (1.6 pints) chicken or vegetable stock
125 g (4 oz) cooked chicken, chopped
25 g (1 oz) Parmesan cheese, grated
Handful of fresh chives or parsley, if available

To balance the meal, add fresh fruit for dessert.

1 Heat the olive oil in a large saucepan.

2 Sauté the onion and peppers over a moderate heat for about 7 minutes.

3 Add the rice and cook for 2–3 mins until the rice is translucent. Add the stock and bring to the boil, partially cover with a lid, and simmer for 12–15 minutes until the rice is tender and the liquid has been absorbed. Add a little more stock if the risotto becomes dry.

4 Add the chicken and half the Parmesan. Heat through for a few minutes.

5 Serve topped with the remaining Parmesan and herbs.

MAIN MEALS

FISH RISOTTO

Makes 4 servings

2 tbsp (30 ml) olive oil
I onion, chopped
175 g (6 oz) long-grain
or Arborio rice
600 ml (I pint) vegetable
stock*
I bay leaf
350 g (12 oz) frozen or smoked
haddock fillet, thawed
200 g (7 oz) frozen peas
Salt and freshly ground black pepper
*Alternatively, use 2 tsp Swiss
vegetable bouillon powder, or I
vegetable stock cube dissolved in 600
ml (I pint) water

To balance the meal, add fresh tomatoes or salad.

1 Heat the olive oil in a large saucepan.
Add the rice and onion
and sauté for 2–3 minutes until the rice
is translucent.

2 Place the rice in a large pan with the
stock and add the bay leaf. Bring to the
boil. Cover and simmer for 15 minutes.

3 Add the haddock and peas and continue
cooking for a further 5 minutes until the
liquid has been absorbed and the fish
flakes easily. Roughly break up the fish
and stir the rice mixture to distribute
evenly.

FISH CAKES

All fish is rich in protein and important minerals. Salmon, in particular, is rich in the essential omega-3 fatty acids, important for brain development and physical activity.

Makes 4 large or 8 small fish cakes

450 g (I lb) potatoes,
peeled
450 g (I lb) salmon or
cod fillet, skinned
60 g (2 oz) butter
4 tbsp (60 ml) milk
I tbsp (15 ml) fresh parsley, chopped
Salt and freshly ground black pepper

To balance the meal, add carrots and peas.

1 Cut the potatoes into quarters and boil
for 15 minutes until soft. Drain.

2 Meanwhile, poach the fish in water for
10 minutes. Drain and flake the fish,
carefully removing all the bones.

3 Mash the potatoes with the butter, milk,
parsley and salt and pepper. Mix in the
flaked fish. Shape into 4 or 8 cakes.

4 Shallow fry in olive oil for a few minutes
on each side. Drain on kitchen paper.

BEAN AND TUNA SALAD

The beans provide protein, B vitamins, iron and fibre.

Makes 4 servings

To balance the meal, add cooked pasta shapes.

1 tin (420g) cannelini or butter beans, drained

2 tomatoes, cubed

1 tin (100 g) tuna in brine, drained and flaked

125 g (4 oz) green beans, cooked and cooled

1 tbsp (15 ml) red wine vinegar

2 tbsp (30 ml) olive oil

Handful of fresh herbs: chives, parsley

1 Combine the tinned beans, tomatoes, tuna and green beans in a bowl.

2 Mix together the vinegar, oil and herbs and combine with the salad.

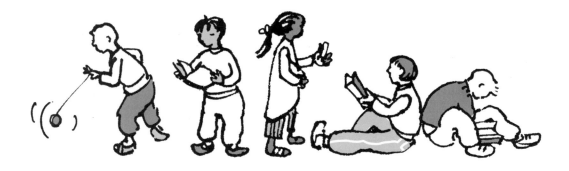

15 MEATLESS MAIN MEALS

VEGETARIAN SPAGHETTI BOLOGNESE

Lentils are substituted for the meat in the Bolognese sauce. They provide plenty of protein, iron, fibre and B vitamins and make a super-tasty main course.

Makes 4 servings

1 tbsp (15 ml) olive oil
1 onion, chopped
2 carrots, grated
1 large courgette, finely chopped
1 tin (400g) chopped tomatoes
1 tin (420g) green lentils (or 125 g (4 oz) dried lentils, soaked and cooked)
1 tsp (5 ml) dried mixed herbs
175 g (6 oz) spaghetti (adjust quantity depending on appetite)
1 tbsp (15 ml) olive oil
2 tbsp (30 ml) Parmesan cheese, grated

To balance the meal, add fresh fruit.

1 Heat the olive oil in a large frying pan. Add the vegetables, stirring often for about 5 minutes, until softened.

2 Add the tomatoes, lentils and herbs. Cook for a further 5–10 minutes until the sauce thickens slightly.

3 Meanwhile, cook the spaghetti in boiling water according to the directions on the packet. Drain and toss in a little olive oil.

4 Divide the spaghetti between 4 bowls. Spoon over the Bolognese sauce and sprinkle on the Parmesan cheese.

PASTA SHELLS WITH TOMATO AND PEPPERS

This is one of the quickest stand-by dishes in my house! You can add other vegetables, such as mushrooms, courgettes or green beans to the tomato sauce instead of peppers.

Makes 4 servings

1 tbsp (15 ml) olive oil
1 onion, chopped
2 garlic cloves, crushed
1 red or green pepper, chopped
1 tin (400g) chopped tomatoes
2 tbsp (30 ml) tomato puree
1 tsp (5 ml) dried basil
Salt and freshly ground black pepper
Pinch of sugar
175 g (6 oz) pasta shells (adjust quantity depending on appetite)
85 g (3 oz) Cheddar cheese, grated

To balance the meal, add broccoli or Brussels sprouts.

1 Heat the olive oil in a large frying pan. Add the onions, garlic and peppers and sauté for 5 minutes or until the vegetables have softened.

2 Add the tomatoes, tomato puree, basil, salt, pepper and sugar. Cook for 5 minutes or until the sauce thickens slightly.

3 Meanwhile, cook the pasta shells in boiling water according to the directions on the packet. Drain.

4 Combine the sauce with the pasta. Spoon into 4 dishes and sprinkle over the cheese.

MARVELLOUS MACARONI CHEESE

Macaroni cheese is popular with most children. Here's a more nutritious version with peas and mushrooms but it also works well with broad beans, carrots and red kidney beans

Makes 4 servings

175 g (6 oz) macaroni (adjust quantity depending on appetite)
60 g (2 oz) frozen peas
25 g (1 oz) butter
60 g (2 oz) button mushrooms, sliced
25 g (1 oz) cornflour
300 ml (½ pint) milk (full-fat or semi-skimmed)
½ teaspoon Dijon mustard
85g (3oz) mature Cheddar grated
Freshly ground black pepper

To balance the meal, add green beans

1 Pre-heat the oven to 200°C/ 400°F/ gas mark 6.

2 Cook the macaroni in boiling water according to the packet, adding the frozen peas during the last 3 minutes of cooking time. Drain.

3 Heat the butter in a pan. Add the mushrooms and sauté for 2 minutes.

4 Blend the cornflour with a little of the milk in a jug. Gradually add the remainder of the milk.

5 Gradually add the milk to the mushrooms in the pan, stirring continuously until the sauce just reaches the boil and has thickened.

6 Remove from the heat, stir in mustard, half the cheese and pepper to taste.

7 Stir in the macaroni and peas. Spoon into an ovenproof dish, sprinkle the remaining cheese over the top and bake for 15–20 minutes until the top is bubbling and golden.

MEATLESS
MAIN MEALS

PENNE WITH CHEESE AND BROCCOLI

Broccoli is full of vitamin C, folate and other powerful antioxidants. This recipe is a tasty way of getting your children to eat it!

Makes 4 servings

175 g (6 oz) penne pasta (adjust quantity depending on appetite)
225 g (8 oz) broccoli florets
1 tbsp (15 ml) olive oil
1 large onion, sliced
1 tbsp (15 ml) cornflour
300 ml (½ pint) milk
60 g (2 oz) mature Cheddar cheese

To balance the meal, add carrots or sliced tomatoes.

1 Cook the pasta in boiling water according to the directions on the packet, adding the broccoli during the last 3 minutes of cooking time. Drain.

2 In a non-stick pan, sauté the onion in the olive oil for 5 minutes until softened.

3 Blend the cornflour with a little of the milk in a jug. Gradually add the remainder of the milk. Slowly add to the onion, stirring continuously until the sauce has thickened. Stir in the cheese.

4 Combine with the pasta and broccoli.

CHICKPEA AND SPINACH PASTA

This is a great way of including spinach in your children's diet. It is rich in iron, folate and vitamin C.

Makes 4 servings

1 tin (410 g) chickpeas, drained and rinsed
½ jar (½ × 440 g) pasta sauce
225 g (8 oz) penne pasta
125 g (4 oz) baby spinach leaves
Salt and freshly ground black pepper
30 g (1 oz) Parmesan cheese, grated
4 tbsp (60 ml) water

To balance the meal, add fresh fruit for dessert.

1 Place the chickpeas in a medium pan with the pasta, sauce together with the water. Bring gently to the boil then turn off the heat and cover.

2 Meanwhile cook the pasta in boiling water according to the directions on the packet. Drain. Stir in the spinach and allow it to wilt.

3 Spoon the pasta into a serving dish and pour the hot pasta sauce and chickpea mixture over the top. Combine together and season with salt and pepper. Top each serving with grated Parmesan.

RED KIDNEY BEAN LASAGNE

This dish is a firm favourite with my children. The combination of pasta, vegetables, red kidney beans and cheese makes it a near-perfect balanced meal.

Makes 4 servings

1 tbsp (15 ml) olive oil
1 onion, chopped
1 red pepper, chopped
60 g (2 oz) mushrooms, chopped
1 courgette, sliced
1 tsp (5 ml) dried basil
Salt and freshly ground black pepper
1 tin (400g) red kidney beans, drained
400 g (14 oz) passata (smooth sieved tomatoes)
85 g (3 oz) mature Cheddar cheese, grated
9 sheets lasagne (no need to pre-cook variety)

To balance the meal, add fresh fruit.

1 Pre-heat the oven to 180°C/ 350°F/ gas mark 4.

2 Heat the oil in a large frying pan. Cook the onion for 3–4 minutes. Add the other vegetables and continue cooking for 2–3 minutes.

3 Add the basil, salt, pepper, red kidney beans and passata. Simmer for 5 minutes until the sauce thickens slightly.

4 Lay a layer of lasagne at the bottom of an oiled baking dish. Cover with one third of the bean mixture. Continue with the layers, finishing with the bean mixture.

5 Sprinkle over the Cheddar and bake for 30 minutes until bubbling and golden.

CRISPY VEGETABLE GRATIN

This recipe is a super way of serving vegetables to children who do not like them plain.

Makes 4 servings

225 g (8 oz) cauliflower, cut into florets
225 g (8 oz) broccoli, cut into florets
30 g (1 oz) butter or margarine
300 ml (½ pint) milk (full-fat or semi-skimmed)
1 tbsp (15 ml) cornflour
1 tsp (5 ml) Dijon mustard
85 g (3 oz) mature Cheddar cheese, grated
2 tbsp (30 ml) flaked almonds or sesame seeds

To balance the meal, add jacket or boiled potatoes.

1 Cook the cauliflower and broccoli in a little fast-boiling water for 5 minutes. Drain and reserve the liquid.

2 Melt the butter in a saucepan.

3 Blend the cornflour with a little of the milk. Gradually add the remaining milk. Add to the melted butter, stirring constantly over a low heat, until the sauce thickens. Mix in the mustard and half of the cheese.

4 Arrange the vegetables in a baking dish and pour over the sauce. Sprinkle with the remaining cheese and almonds or sesame seeds.

5 Place under a hot grill until golden brown.

BEAN BURRITOS

These tasty burritos are a new spin on pancakes, always popular with children. The bean filling is high in protein, fibre and iron.

Makes 4 burritos

1 tbsp (15 ml) olive oil
1 onion, chopped
1 clove of garlic, crushed
1 tbsp (15 ml) taco seasoning mix (according to taste)
1 tin (420 g) pinto or red kidney beans (or use 175 g/6 oz dried beans, soaked, cooked and drained)
200 g (½ 400 g tin) chopped tomatoes or 200 g (7 oz) salsa
4 small soft wheat tortillas
225 g (8 oz) passata with herbs or garlic
60 g (2 oz) grated mature Cheddar cheese, grated

To balance the meal, add a green vegetable or salad.

1 Pre-heat the oven to 160°C/ 350°F/ gas mark 4.

2 Heat the oil in a large frying pan. Sauté the onion and garlic for 5 minutes.

3 Add the taco seasoning mix, kidney beans and chopped tomatoes or salsa to the pan. Roughly mash the beans and cook for a further 3 minutes until the sauce has thickened a little.

4 Spread one quarter of the mixture over each tortilla. Roll up and place seam-side down in an oiled baking dish.

5 Spoon the passata over the tortillas; sprinkle over the cheese.

6 Cover with foil and bake for 20–30 minutes until golden.

CHICKPEA HOTPOT

This one-pot dish is quick and easy to prepare and makes a perfect midweek supper. Chickpeas are rich in protein, iron and zinc. Use any variety of tinned beans in place of the chickpeas if you wish.

Makes 4 servings

1 tbsp (15 ml) olive oil
1 onion, chopped
1 garlic clove, crushed
2 courgettes, sliced
1 tsp (5 ml) dried mixed herbs
1 tin (400g) chopped tomatoes
1 tin (420 g) chick peas, drained
1 vegetable stock cube
40 g (1½ oz) Cheddar cheese, grated

To balance the meal, add fresh fruit for dessert.

1 Heat the oil in a large pan and sauté the onion and garlic for 3–4 minutes until softened. Add the courgettes and cook for a further 2 minutes.

2 Add the herbs, tomatoes, chickpeas and crumbled stock cube. Stir well and bring to the boil. Simmer for further 10 minutes, adding a little water if necessary.

3 Spoon in to a baking dish, sprinkle with grated cheese.

4 Melt the cheese under a hot grill until the cheese is bubbling.

RED LENTIL DAHL

Red lentils are a superb source of protein, iron, fibre and B vitamins. This mildly spiced dahl will appeal to children.

Makes 4 servings

To balance the meal, add boiled rice and a green vegetable.

1 tbsp (15 ml) sunflower oil
1 onion, chopped
1 garlic clove, crushed
½ tsp (5 ml) ground cumin
1 tsp (5 ml) ground coriander
½ tsp turmeric
175 g (6oz) red lentils
850 ml (1½ pints) water
Salt and freshly ground black pepper

1 Heat the oil in a large pan and fry the onion for about 5 minutes. Add the garlic and spices and fry for a further 2 minutes.
2 Add the lentils and water and bring to the boil. Cover and simmer for about 30 minutes.
3 Season with salt and pepper to taste.

BUTTER BEAN AND LEEK SUPPER

This nutritious combination of pulses and vegetables is easy to prepare. You can add other vegetables, such as mushrooms or peppers, to make it a more substantial dish.

Makes 4 servings

To balance the meal, add new potatoes and grated cheese.

1 tbsp (15 ml) olive oil
2 leeks, sliced
1 tin (400g) chopped tomatoes
1 tin (420g) butter beans, drained
150 ml (¼ pint) vegetable stock*
*Alternatively, use ½ tsp (2.5 ml) Swiss vegetable bouillon powder or ¼ vegetable stock cube dissolved in 150 ml (¼ pint) water

1 Sauté the leeks in the olive oil for about 5 minutes until the leeks are almost soft.
2 Add the remaining ingredients, stir and bring to the boil. Simmer for a further 10–15 minutes or until the sauce has thickened.

MEATLESS MAIN MEALS

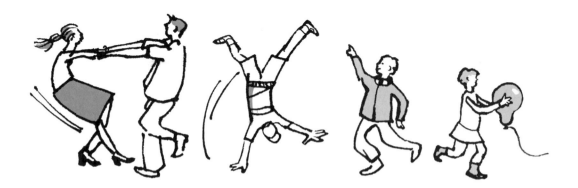

VEGETABLE KORMA

Traditional kormas are made with cream. This recipe uses cashew nuts and milk in place of the cream and is a delicious way of introducing children to new flavours. Vary the vegetables according to what you have available.

Makes 4 servings

150 ml (¼ pint) milk
40 g (1½ oz) cashew nut pieces
1 tbsp (15 ml) sunflower oil
1 onion, sliced
½ tsp (2½ ml) of each: ground cumin, garam masala and turmeric
(Alternatively use 2 tsp (10 ml) mild curry powder)
1 garlic clove, crushed
125 g (4 oz) cauliflower florets
1 courgette, sliced
60 g (2 oz) mushrooms
85 g (3 oz) baby corn cobs
Salt to taste

To balance the meal, add mini naan breads or boiled rice.

1 Bring the milk to the boil, remove from the heat and add the cashews. Leave to soak for 15 minutes, then purée until smooth using a hand blender or food processor.

2 Heat the oil in a large pan and sauté the onion for 5 minutes.

3 Add the spices and the garlic and continue cooking for 2 minutes.

4 Add the vegetables, cover and simmer for 10 minutes or until the vegetables are just tender. Season with the salt.

5 Stir in the cashew 'cream' and simmer for a further 2 minutes.

VEGETABLE RICE FEAST

This glorious medley of vegetables and rice is a great way of adding vegetables to children's diets. The peas and pine nuts add protein to the dish.

Makes 4 servings

1 tbsp (15 ml) olive oil
1 onion, chopped
1 garlic clove, crushed
2 celery sticks, chopped
1 red or yellow pepper, chopped
175 g (6 oz) rice (adjust the quantity according to children's appetite)
450 ml (¾ pint) vegetable stock*
125 g (4 oz) frozen peas
Salt and freshly ground black pepper to taste
30 g (1 oz) pine nuts
*Alternatively, use 1½ tsp (7.5 ml) Swiss vegetable bouillon, or 1 stock cube dissolved in 450 ml (¾ pint) water

To balance the meal, add yoghurt for dessert.

1 Heat the oil in a large pan and sauté the onion, garlic, celery and pepper for 5 minutes.

2 Add the rice and stir for another 2–3 minutes.

3 Add the stock, bring to the boil, then simmer for 15–20 minutes until the liquid has been absorbed.

4 Add the peas during the last 3 minutes of cooking, season to taste and heat through for a few more minutes. Serve sprinkled with the pine nuts.

COUS COUS WITH NUTS AND VEGETABLES

Cous cous is easy to prepare and children enjoy its soft texture. Mix it with vegetables and nuts and it makes a delicious balanced meal.

Makes 4 servings

175 g (6 oz) cous cous
450 ml (¾ pint) vegetable stock*
1 tbsp (15 ml) olive oil
1 onion, chopped
1 red pepper, chopped
85 g (3 oz) baby corn cobs
1 carrot, diced
60 g (2 oz) dates, chopped (optional)
60 g (2 oz) flaked toasted almonds
*Alternatively, use 1½ tsp (7.5 ml) Swiss vegetable bouillon or 1 stock cube dissolved in 450 ml (¾ pint) water

To balance the meal, add fruit and custard for dessert.

1 Bring the stock to the boil then remove from the heat. Pour over the cous cous and leave to stand for 15 minutes until all the liquid has been absorbed.

2 Meanwhile heat the oil in a pan and sauté the onion for 5 minutes. Add the vegetables and continue cooking for about 7–10 minutes or until the vegetables are tender-crisp (not soft).

3 Fluff the cous cous with a fork and stir in the vegetables, almonds and dates, if using.

POTATO AND CHEESE PIE

This simple dish of potatoes and cheese is, in fact, a childhood favourite of mine. My children are equally fond of it. Layer sliced leeks or broccoli florets with the cheese to increase the vegetable content.

Makes 4 servings

450 g (1 lb) potatoes
300 ml (½ pint) milk
60 g (2oz) grated cheese
1 onion, thinly sliced
2 large tomatoes, sliced
2 eggs
Salt and freshly ground black pepper

To balance the meal, add baked beans and a green vegetable.

1 Pre-heat the oven to 200°C/ 400°F/ gas mark 6.

2 Peel and thinly slice the potatoes. Arrange layers of potato, cheese, onion and tomatoes in a shallow baking dish, finishing with cheese.

3 Beat the eggs with the milk, season with salt and pepper then pour over the potatoes.

4 Cover with foil and bake for 45–60 minutes until the potatoes are tender and the top golden brown.

SALADS

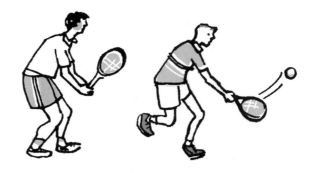

PERFECT SALAD

This salad is an almost perfectly balanced meal. It provides every vitamin and mineral, including calcium from the nuts and yoghurt, protein from the red kidney beans and nuts, and carbohydrate from the pasta. To add variety to the salad leaves use watercress, rocket, endive or baby spinach where available.

Makes 4 servings

125 g (4 oz) pasta shells
½ red pepper
½ yellow pepper
60 g (2 oz) toasted flaked almonds, cashews or peanuts
60 g (2 oz) raisins
125 g (4 oz) cooked or canned red kidney beans
2 tomatoes, sliced
1 apple, sliced
Mixed salad leaves
For the dressing:
3 tbsp (45 ml) plain yoghurt or low-fat mayonnaise
1 tbsp (15 ml) salad cream

To balance the meal, add fresh fruit for dessert.

1 Cook the pasta shells according to directions on the packet. Drain.

2 Mix the pasta with the peppers, nuts, raisins, beans, tomatoes and apple slices.

3 Arrange the salad leaves on a serving dish. Pile the pasta mixture on top.

4 Mix the dressing ingredients together and pour over the salad.

POTATO SALAD

This is an excellent portable snack or lunch. New potatoes contain twice as much vitamin C as old potatoes. You can add extra vegetables such as spring onions and radishes.

Makes 4 servings

450 g (1 lb) new or old potatoes, cut into small chunks (no need to peel)
1 tablespoon (15 ml) each of fresh chopped mint and parsley
15 cm (6 in) piece cucumber, diced
1 tbsp (15 ml) plain yoghurt
1 tbsp (15 ml) salad cream (or mayonnaise)
Freshly ground black pepper

To balance the meal, add boiled eggs or cottage cheese and some vegetable crudités.

1 Boil the potatoes in a little fast-boiling water for 5–7 minutes until just tender. Drain.
2 Combine the remaining ingredients together. Toss in the cooled potatoes and optional ingredients.

RICE AND SWEETCORN SALAD

This salad is easy to prepare and the peppers are a great source of vitamin C. The almonds provide protein and calcium.

Makes 4 servings

175 g (6 oz) rice (adjust the quantity according to your children's appetite)
2 red peppers, chopped
125 g (4 oz) sultanas
60 g (2 oz) split almonds, roughly chopped
1 tin (225 g (8 oz)) sweetcorn, drained

To balance the meal, add red kidney beans or hummus.

1 Cook the rice according to directions on the packet. Drain if necessary, rinse in cold water and drain again.
2 Place the cooled rice in a large bowl and combine with the remaining ingredients.

SALADS

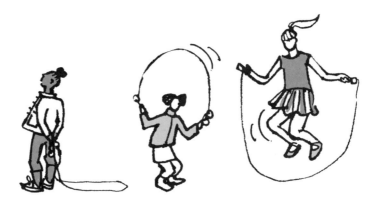

COLESLAW

Children love the crunchiness of shredded cabbage combined with the smooth creaminess of mayonnaise. Raw cabbage is packed with vitamin C and, though mayonnaise is high in fat, it's mostly the healthly unsaturated kind. Add any of the optional ingredients listed below to the basic recipe — it's a great way of getting your children to eat extra raw vegetables.

Makes 4 servings

125 ml (4 fl oz) low-fat mayonnaise
1 small head of white or green cabbage, finely shredded
1 large carrot, peeled and grated
Salt and freshly ground black pepper, to taste

1 Place the cabbage and carrots in a large bowl and stir in just enough mayonnaise to moisten the vegetables. Season with salt and pepper.

2 Add any of the following:

- Chopped fresh parsley or chives
- Pineapple chunks
- Finely chopped onions or spring onions
- Finely chopped peppers
- Red cabbage
- Brocolli
- Cauliflower
- Raisins
- Cashews
- Beetroot
- Sunflower seeds
- Toasted pumpkin seeds
- Grated eating apple
- Celery
- Chicory
- Celeriac

SALAD DRESSINGS

Most children reach for salad cream when confronted with raw salads. However, most shop-bought salad dressings are high in salt and contain artificial additives. Here are some quick and healthy alternatives that require no or very little preparation.

- A drizzle of balsamic vinegar
- A squeeze of lemon juice
- Plain yoghurt mixed with an equal quantity of salad cream
- Greek yoghurt mixed with a squeeze of lemon juice and chopped fresh parsley

Olive oil and vinegar dressing

3 tbsp (45 ml) olive oil
1 tbsp (15 ml) white wine vinegar or lemon juice
Pinch of sugar
Pinch of salt
Freshly ground black pepper to taste

Shake the ingredients together in a screw-top jar.

Serving Suggestion: As a dressing for leafy salads, cucumber salad and bean salads.

Herb Dressing

60 ml (2 fl oz) cider vinegar
2 tbsp (30 ml) orange juice
1 tbsp (15 ml) olive oil
1 garlic clove, crushed
1 tbsp (15 ml) chopped fresh parsley or oregano

Place the ingredients in a screw top jar and shake well to combine.

Serving Suggestion: As a dressing for lettuce and other leaf salads, coleslaw or with cooked green vegetables such as broccoli and green beans.

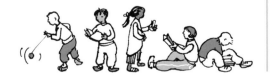

SUPER SOUPS

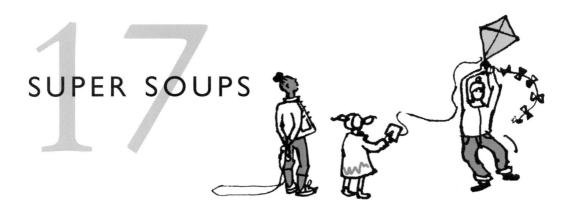

POTATO SOUP

This is an ideal main meal soup as it is rich in energy-giving carbohydrate and the milk also provides protein and calcium. Sweet potatoes provide beta-carotene and omega-3 fatty acids, essential for brain development.

Makes 4 servings

2 tbsp (30 ml) olive oil
1 onion, chopped
3 medium potatoes, scrubbed and chopped into chunks
1 sweet potato, peeled and chopped into chunks
2 teaspoons (10 ml) Swiss vegetable bouillon powder*
450 ml (¾ pint) water
600 ml (1 pint) skimmed milk
Freshly ground black pepper
Handful of chopped fresh parsley or thyme if available
* Alternatively, use 1 vegetable stock cube

To balance the meal, add grated cheese; fresh fruit for dessert.

1 Heat the oil in a large heavy-bottomed saucepan. Cook the onion on a low heat for 5 minutes until it becomes transparent.
2 Add the potatoes, stir and cook on a low heat for 2 minutes.
3 Add the vegetable bouillon powder and the water. Bring to the boil and simmer for about 20 minutes until the potatoes are soft.
4 Remove from the heat and mash or liquidise with the milk.
5 Return to the saucepan, add some freshly ground black pepper and fresh herbs. Heat through until just hot.

REAL TOMATO SOUP

Tomato soup is a firm favourite with children. It's also a great way of hiding extra vegetables, such as carrots and red peppers. This soup is packed with vitamin C, beta-carotene and the powerful antioxidant lycopene.

Makes 4 servings

2 tbsp (30 ml) olive oil
1 onion, chopped
1 large carrot, grated
1 red pepper, chopped
1 large potato, peeled and cubed
2 garlic cloves, crushed
2 tsp (10 ml) Swiss vegetable bouillon powder*
1 tin (400 g) chopped tomatoes
750 ml (1¼ pints) water
1 tsp (5 ml) sugar
Freshly ground black pepper
* Alternatively, use 1 vegetable stock cube

To balance the meal, add grated cheese and crusty wholemeal bread.

1 Sauté the onion in the oil for 2–3 minutes in a large saucepan. Add the carrot, red pepper, potato and garlic and cook for a further 5 minutes.

2 Add the vegetable bouillon powder, tomatoes, water and sugar. Simmer for about 20 minutes or until the vegetables are soft.

3 Liquidise the soup using a hand blender or food processor and season with the black pepper.

BROCCOLI AND CHEESE SOUP

This simple soup makes a nutritionally complete meal and is an ingenious way to get children to eat broccoli. It is rich in protein, fibre, vitamin C and complex carbohydrate.

Makes 4 servings

1 onion, chopped
300 g (10 oz) broccoli florets
450 ml (¾ pint) vegetable stock*
450 ml (¾ pint) semi-skimmed milk
60 g (2 oz) mature Cheddar cheese, grated
Pinch of freshly grated nutmeg (optional)
Salt and freshly ground black pepper
*Alternatively, use 1½ tsp (7.5 ml) Swiss vegetable bouillon powder or 1 vegetable stock cube dissolved in 450 ml (¾ pint) water

To balance the meal, add crusty wholemeal rolls.

1 Place the onion, broccoli and vegetable stock in a saucepan. Bring to the boil and simmer for about 15 minutes or until the vegetables are soft.

2 Liquidise the soup using a hand blender or food processor.

3 Return to the saucepan with the milk. Heat until almost at boiling point.

4 Add the grated Cheddar cheese, stirring until it melts.

BUTTERNUT SQUASH SOUP

This is my children's favourite soup. Butternut squash is very rich in beta-carotene and makes a wonderful soup. Its subtle sweetness appeals to children. You can substitute pumpkin or other varieties of squash for the butternut squash if you wish.

Makes 4 servings

2 tbsp (30 ml) olive oil
1 onion, chopped
450 g (1 lb) butternut squash, peeled and chopped
1 large carrot, sliced
1 medium potato, peeled and chopped
2 tsp (10 ml) Swiss vegetable bouillon powder*
900 ml (1½ pints) water
1 tsp (5 ml) grated fresh ginger (or ½ teaspoon (5 ml) ground ginger)
Freshly ground black pepper
*Alternatively, use 1 vegetable stock cube

To balance the meal, add grated cheese and wholemeal bread.

1 Sauté the onion in the olive oil for about 5 minutes until transparent.

2 Add the butternut squash, carrot and potato and cook for a further 2–3 minutes.

3 Add the vegetable bouillon powder and water and bring to the boil. Turn down the heat and simmer for 20 minutes or until the vegetables are tender.

4 Remove from the heat. Liquidise the soup using a hand blender or food processor.

5 Season with pepper.

CARROT SOUP

This soup is inexpensive and simple to make, and packed with the antioxidant beta-carotene.

Makes 4 servings

2 tbsp (30 ml) olive oil
1 onion, chopped
1 clove of garlic, crushed
675 g (1½ lb) carrots, sliced
900 ml (1½ pints) vegetable stock*
Salt and freshly ground black pepper
1–2 tablespoons fresh coriander, chopped (optional)
*Alternatively, use 3 tsp (15 ml) Swiss vegetable bouillon or 1½ vegetable stock cubes in 900 ml (1½ pints) water

To balance the meal, add a swirl of plain yoghurt or grated cheese and crusty wholemeal rolls.

1 Sauté the onion and garlic in the olive oil for 5 minutes in a large saucepan.

2 Add the carrots and continue cooking for a further 2 minutes.

3 Add the stock and bring to the boil, then reduce the heat and simmer for 15 minutes or until the carrots are tender.

4 Season with the salt and pepper and add the fresh coriander.

5 Liquidise using a hand blender or food processor.

SUPER SOUPS

153

VEGETABLE AND PASTA SOUP

This soup is ideal for hiding vegetables your children may not normally choose to eat on their own. Vary the vegetables according to what you have available.

Makes 4–6 servings
2 tbsp (30 ml) olive oil
1 onion, chopped
1 garlic clove, crushed
1 red pepper, chopped
1 litre (1¾ pints) vegetable stock*
1 tin (400 g) chopped tomatoes
2 large carrots, chopped
125 g (4 oz) cauliflower
2 medium potatoes, peeled and cubed
85 g (3 oz) small pasta shapes
125 g (4 oz) frozen peas
Salt and freshly ground black pepper
*Alternatively, use 3 tsp (15 ml) Swiss bouillon or 2 vegetable stock cubes plus 1 litre (1¾ pints) water

To balance the meal, add grated cheese.

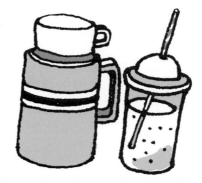

1 Sauté the onion, garlic and red pepper in the olive oil for 5 minutes.

2 Add the other vegetables, except the peas, and cook for a further 2 minutes. Add the vegetable stock, bring to the boil and simmer for about 20 minutes.

3 Add the pasta shapes and frozen peas about 10 minutes before the end of the cooking time.

4 Serve. Alternatively, for a chunky thick soup, liquidise half the soup after step 2 and return to the pan.

FAST FOOD

HOMEMADE CHICKEN NUGGETS

These homemade chicken nuggets are far healthier than the ready-bought and takeaway versions. The wheat germ used for the coating provides essential B vitamins (thiamin and niacin), iron and zinc. They are baked rather than fried, reducing the fat content and the need for artificial flavour enhancers.

Makes 4 servings

3 chicken breasts, boneless, skinned
85 g (3 oz) wheat germ
½ teaspoon (2.5 ml) salt
½ teaspoon (1.25 ml) garlic powder
Freshly ground black pepper
90 ml (3 fl oz) water
1 egg white

To balance the meal, add Potato Wedges (page 162), carrots and peas.

1 Pre-heat the oven to 200°C/ 400°F/ gas mark 6.
2 Cut the chicken breasts into small chunks.
3 Combine the wheat germ, salt, garlic powder and a little pepper. Place the mixture in a large plastic bag.
4 Combine the water and egg white in a bowl. Dip the chicken pieces into the egg mixture, and then drop into the plastic bag. Shake until the chicken is thoroughly coated.
5 Place the coated chicken pieces on an oiled baking tray. Bake for 10–15 minutes or until tender and golden brown, turning once midway through cooking.

CHICKEN BURGERS

These are a healthy alternative to beefburgers due to their lower fat content. Unlike traditional burgers, they are dry-fried so they don't absorb lots of oil.

Makes 4 burgers

1 onion, finely chopped
1 stick celery, finely chopped
1 clove garlic, crushed
2 tbsp (30 ml) olive oil
2 chicken breasts, skinless and boneless
2 tbsp (30 ml) fresh parsley, chopped (or 1 tbsp (15 ml) dried parsley)
60 g (2 oz) fresh breadcrumbs
Salt and freshly ground black pepper
1 egg yolk
Flour for coating

To balance the meal, add a wholemeal bap, shredded lettuce, sliced tomatoes, onion rings and a little salsa or relish.

1 Sauté the onion, celery and garlic in the olive oil for 5 minutes. Meanwhile mince or finely chop the chicken in a food processor.

2 Combine the onion mixture, chicken, parsley and breadcrumbs in a bowl. Season with salt and pepper and bind the mixture together with the egg yolk.

3 Form into 4 burgers, roll in flour and dry-fry in a non-stick pan over a medium heat until golden and cooked through, turning halfway through (about 5–6 minutes each side).

SPICY BEAN BURGERS

This is a great vegetarian treat that even my children's non-vegetarian friends enjoy. The beans are a good source of protein, iron and B vitamins, but you can use other beans, such as butter beans, flageolet or cannelloni beans instead. You can hide lots of vegetables in the burgers, too.

Makes 8 small or 4 large burgers

2 tins (400 g × 2) red kidney beans
1 tbsp (15 ml) olive oil
1 onion, chopped
1 clove of garlic, crushed
1 celery stick, chopped
1 carrot, finely grated
1 green pepper, chopped
½ tsp (2.5 ml) ground cumin
½ tsp (2.5 ml) ground coriander
1 tbsp (15 ml) tomato purée
1 tbsp fresh coriander, chopped (optional)
1 egg
60 g (2 oz) dried breadcrumbs
60 g (2 oz) Cheddar cheese, grated
Salt and freshly ground black pepper

To balance the meal, add a wholemeal bap, lettuce, sliced tomatoes, onion rings and salsa.

1 Pre-heat oven to 200°C/400°F/gas mark 6

2 Drain then mash the beans in a bowl.

3 Heat the oil in a frying pan and sauté the onion for 3–4 mins until transparent. Add the garlic, celery, carrot, green pepper, spices and cook for a further 5 mins.

4 Add the mashed beans, tomato purée, egg, breadcrumbs and cheese. Mix together, then shape into 8 small/4 large burgers.

5 Place on an oiled baking tray. Bake in the oven for 25 mins until golden and crisp.

LEAN MEAT BURGERS

These homemade meat burgers are made with lean mince and cooked without extra oil. This means they are low in fat—and at least you know exactly what's in them!

Makes 8 small or 4 large burgers

350 g (12 oz) extra lean minced meat (beef, turkey, pork)
60 g (2 oz) dried breadcrumbs
3 tbsp (45 ml) water
1 small onion, chopped
2 tbsp (30 ml) fresh sage or parsley, chopped (or 1 tbsp (15 ml) dried)
Freshly ground black pepper

To balance the meal, add a wholemeal bap, shredded lettuce, sliced tomatoes, relish or salsa and plenty of salad.

1 Place the minced meat, breadcrumbs, water, onion, herbs and pepper in a bowl. Mix well to combine.

2 Divide the mixture into 4 or 8 balls and flatten into burgers. Dry fry in a hot non-stick pan for 3–4 minutes each side. Alternatively, place the burgers on a baking sheet and cook in the oven at 200°C/ 400°F/ gas mark 6 for 10–15 minutes depending on the size of the burgers. Test by inserting a skewer into the middle of a burger—there should be no trace of pink in the meat and the juices should run clear.

SPICY LENTIL BURGERS

These tasty burgers are made with red lentils, a terrific source of protein, iron and fibre. They are oven-baked using only a little oil.

Makes 8 small or 4 large burgers

1 tbsp (15 ml) olive oil
1 onion, finely chopped
1–2 tsp (5–10 ml) curry powder (depending on your children's tastes)
175 g (6 oz) red lentils (dried, no need to soak)
600 ml (1 pint) vegetable stock
125 g (4 oz) fresh wholemeal breadcrumbs
Salt and freshly ground black pepper to taste
A little oil for brushing

To balance the meal, add a wholemeal bap or jacket potato, shredded lettuce, sliced tomatoes, onion rings and a little salsa or relish.

1 Pre-heat the oven to 200°C/ 400°F/ gas mark 6.

2 Heat the olive oil in a large pan and sauté the onion until softened. Stir in the curry powder and cook for a further 2 minutes.

3 Add the lentils and stock. Bring to the boil and simmer for 20–25 minutes.

4 Allow to cool slightly then mix in the breadcrumbs. Shape into 4 or 8 burgers.

5 Place on a lightly oiled baking tray and brush each burger with a little oil.

6 Bake for 7–10 minutes until golden and firm.

NUT BURGERS

These delicious burgers are a real hit with my children. Nuts are a terrific source of essential fats, protein, iron, zinc and B vitamins. You can substitute other types of nuts, such as almonds, hazelnuts or peanuts for the cashews if you wish.

Makes 4 large or 8 small burgers

To balance the meal, add mashed potato, carrots and peas.

    I onion, chopped
    I garlic clove, crushed
    ½ red pepper
    I tbsp (15 ml) rapeseed oil
    I tsp (5 ml) dried mixed herbs
    I tbsp (15 ml) wholemeal flour
    150 ml (5 fl oz) water
    ½ vegetable stock cube
    225 g (8 oz) cashew nuts
    125 g (4 oz) fresh wholemeal
    breadcrumbs
    Salt and freshly ground black pepper
    A little olive oil for brushing

1 Pre-heat the oven to 200°C/ 400°F/ gas mark 6.

2 Sauté the onion, garlic and red pepper in the oil for 5 minutes until translucent. Add the herbs and flour and continue cooking for a further 2 minutes.

3 Stir in the water and stock cube and continue stirring until the sauce has thickened.

4 Grind the cashews in a food processor then add with the breadcrumbs to the sauce. Season with salt and pepper to taste. Allow to cool slightly.

5 Shape into 4–8 burgers and arrange on an oiled baking tray. Brush lightly with a little olive oil. Bake in the oven for 15–20 minutes until golden and crisp on the outside.

TOMATO SALSA

Tomato salsa makes a great accompaniment to tacos, grilled chicken, and meat or vegetarian burgers. It also enlivens steamed or roasted vegetables, scrambled eggs and cheese on toast.

Makes 4 servings

    2 large ripe tomatoes or 4 ripe plum
    tomatoes, deseeded and finely diced
    1–2 tbsp (15–30 ml) chopped fresh
    parsley or coriander
    I tsp (5 ml) finely chopped fresh chilli
    or ½ tsp (2.5 ml) dried chilli flakes (or
    according to your children's taste)
    I small clove of garlic, crushed
    I tbsp (15 ml) olive oil
    2 spring onions, finely chopped
    2 tbsp (30 ml) lemon or lime juice

1 Combine all the ingredients in a bowl.

2 If time permits, chill in the fridge for about an hour before serving.

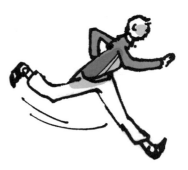

PIZZAS

Making your own pizzas is easy if you have a bread machine. Alternatively, use the quick pizza base recipe, as this doesn't require kneading or proving. It's worth making your own tomato sauce, too, as ready-bought versions contain quite a lot of salt and have that processed flavour we don't want children to get used to.

Makes 1 large pizza

Pizza base:
225 g (8 oz) strong white flour
½ sachet easy-blend yeast
½ tsp salt
175 ml (6 fl oz) warm water
1 tbsp (15 ml) olive oil

1 If making the dough by hand, mix the flour, yeast and salt in a large bowl. Make a well in the centre and add the oil and half the water. Stir with a wooden spoon, gradually adding more liquid until you have a pliable dough. Turn the dough out onto a floured surface and knead for about 5 minutes until you have a smooth and elastic dough. Place the dough in a clean, lightly oiled bowl, cover with a tea towel and leave in a warm place for about 1 hour or until doubled in size.

2 If you are using a bread machine, place the ingredients in the tin and follow the instructions supplied with the machine.

3 Turn out the dough; knead briefly before rolling out on a surface to the desired shape.

4 Transfer to an oiled pizza pan or baking tray and finish shaping by hand. The dough should be approx. 5 mm (¼ in) thick. For a thicker crust, let the dough rise for 30 minutes, otherwise the pizza is now ready for topping and baking.

5 Bake on the top shelf of the oven at 220°C/ 425°F/ gas mark 7 for 15–20 minutes or until the topping is bubbling and the crust is golden brown.

QUICK PIZZA BASE

225 g (8 oz) self-raising white flour
1 tsp (5 ml) baking powder
½ tsp (2.5 ml) salt
40 g (1½ oz) butter or margarine
150 ml (5 fl oz) skimmed milk

1 Mix the flour, baking powder and salt in a bowl.

2 Rub in the butter or margarine until the mixture resembles breadcrumbs.

3 Add the milk, quickly mixing with a fork, just until the mixture comes together.

4 Roll or press the dough into a circle approx 25 cm (10 in) in diameter and transfer onto a baking tray or pizza pan.

5 The base is now ready for topping. Then bake on the top shelf of the oven at 220°C/ 425°F/ gas mark 7 for 15 minutes.

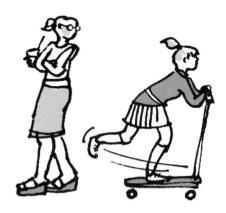

CHEESE AND TOMATO PIZZA

Tomato sauce
1 tbsp (15 ml) olive oil
1 small onion, finely chopped
1 garlic clove, crushed
300 ml (½ pint) passata (smooth sieved tomatoes) or 1 tin (400 g) chopped tomatoes
1 tbsp (15 ml) tomato puree
1 tsp (5 ml) dried basil
½ tsp (2.5 ml) sugar
Pinch of salt and freshly ground black pepper
125 g (4 oz) mozzarella, sliced (or grated Cheddar cheese)

1 Sauté the onion and garlic in the olive oil for 5 minutes until translucent.

2 Add the passata or chopped tomatoes, tomato purée, basil, sugar, salt and pepper. Continue to simmer for 5–10 minutes or until the sauce has thickened a little.

3 Spread the sauce on the pizza base. Scatter over the cheese and any additional toppings from the list below.

4 Bake at 200°C/ 450°F/ gas mark 8 for 15–20 minutes until the cheese is bubbling and golden brown.

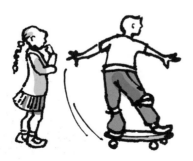

PIZZA TOPPINGS

This is a great opportunity to add extra vegetables to your children's diet. Add any combination of the following:

- tomatoes, sliced
- cherry tomatoes, halved
- red, yellow and green peppers, sliced
- mushrooms, sliced
- sweetcorn
- onion rings
- olives
- courgettes, sliced
- tuna, flaked
- spinach, cooked and drained
- broccoli florets, cooked
- colourful cheeses, e.g. Red Leicester, Double Gloucester
- pineapple
- peas
- leeks, thinly sliced
- baby sweetcorn
- cooked turkey or chicken
- spring onions
- cooked aubergine
- poached egg on top
- salmon (smoked or tinned) and dill
- basil
- oregano

Alternative Pizza Bases

- ready-made pizza base
- English muffin, toasted and split horizontally
- Foccacia bread, halved horizontally
- ciabatta loaf, halved horizontally
- wholemeal or white pitta bread
- french bread, halved horizontally

JACKET POTATOES

Jacket potatoes are excellent fast foods. They are nutritious, delicious and simple to prepare. They provide complex carbohydrates, B vitamins, vitamin C, iron and fibre. Here's how to bake the perfect potato:

1 Wash the potatoes and pierce the skin with a fork.

2 Bake directly on the oven shelf at 220°C/ 425°F/ gas mark 7 for about 1 – 1¼ hours (depending on the size of the potato) or until the flesh is very tender.

3 For a crispy skin, rub lightly in a little olive oil and salt.

Toppings for jacket potatoes

- baked beans
- cheddar cheese
- mozzarella cheese
- plain yoghurt
- half-fat crème fraiche
- salsa
- stir-fried vegetables
- chicken mixed with a little mayonnaise
- hummus
- cottage cheese
- prawns with mayonnaise or salad cream
- ratatouille
- lentil dahl (see page 145)
- tuna mixed with plain yoghurt or mayonnaise
- grilled mushrooms
- chilli con carne (page 161)
- scrambled egg and tomato
- sweetcorn
- bolognese sauce (page 132 — Turkey Bolognese and Lasagne recipes)
- vegetarian bolognese (page 140)
- vegetable korma (page 161)

MIGHTY ROOT MASH

The swede and parsnips give a subtle sweetness, which children will love. They also add extra vitamins to the dish. Extra milk is used in place of the traditional butter to create a soft consistency.

Makes 4 servings

450 g (1 lb) potatoes, peeled and cubed
125 g (4 oz) swede, peeled and cubed
1 parsnip, peeled and cubed
200 ml (7 fl oz) milk
Salt and freshly ground black pepper

To balance the meal, add Chicken Burgers (page 156) or Spicy Bean Burgers (page 156) and a green vegetable.

1 Cook the potato, swede and parsnip in a little fast-boiling water for 15–20 minutes, until tender. Drain.

2 Mash the root vegetables with the milk and seasoning. Add a little extra milk for a softer consistency.

FAST FOOD

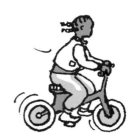

OVEN POTATO WEDGES

These are a real treat for my children. These oven-baked wedges are healthier than chips as they are lower in fat and, with the skins left on, retain much of their vitamin C.

Makes 4 servings

4 medium potatoes, scrubbed (adjust the quantity according to your children's appetite)
4 tsp (20 ml) sunflower or olive oil
Optional: garlic powder; Parmesan cheese; chilli powder

To balance the meal, add baked beans or poached eggs and a green vegetable.

1 Pre-heat the oven to 200°C/ 400°F/ gas mark 6.

2 Cut each potato lengthways, then cut each half into 6 wedges.

3 Place in a baking tin and turn in the oil until each piece is lightly coated.

4 Bake for 35–40 minutes turning occasionally until the potatoes are soft inside and golden brown on the outside.

5 Sprinkle on one of the optional ingredients 5 minutes before the end of cooking.

POTATO TACOS

These tacos are easy to assemble and very nutritious, too. The beans supply protein, iron, B vitamins and fibre and make a tasty partner to the jacket potatoes.

Makes 4 servings

4 potatoes
½ a 420 g tin refried beans, pinto beans or red kidney beans (roughly mashed)
4 tbsp (30 ml) mild taco sauce
125 g (4 oz) Cheddar cheese, grated
4 tbsp (60 ml) plain low-fat yoghurt
Shredded iceberg lettuce
1 tomato, finely chopped

To balance the meal, add pepper strips and cucumber slices.

1 Preheat the oven to 200°C/ 400°F/ gas mark 6.

2 Scrub the potatoes and prick with a fork. Smear with a little oil and salt—this gives a crispy jacket. Bake for about 1 hour.

3 Split the cooked potato and puff it up. Heat the mashed beans. Spoon on the beans and sauce.

4 Top with the grated cheese and yoghurt. Scatter over the lettuce and tomato.

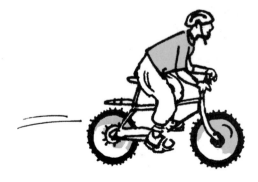

19 AND TO FINISH

RASPBERRY FOOL

Raspberries are full of vitamin C and the fromage frais provides protein and calcium. You may substitute other seasonal fruits such as strawberries, blackberries or, in the winter, mango or stewed apple.

Makes 4 servings

225 g (8 oz) raspberries
225 g (8 oz) low-fat plain fromage frais
1 tbsp (15 ml) clear honey

1 Mash the raspberries lightly with a fork.
2 Mix with the fromage frais and honey. Spoon into 4 bowls.

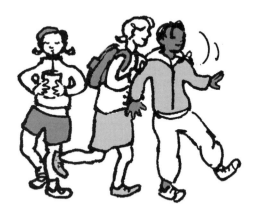

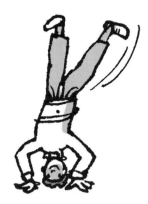

PANCAKES

Pancakes are easy to make and your children will have tremendous fun tossing them! This recipe uses a 50/50 mixture of wholemeal and white flour to boost the vitamin, iron and fibre content. The eggs and milk are good sources of protein and the fruit fillings will provide extra vitamins.

Makes 10–12 pancakes

70 g (2 ½ oz) plain white flour
70 g (2 ½ oz) plain wholemeal flour
2 size 3 eggs
250 ml (8 fl oz) milk (full-fat or semi-skimmed)
A little vegetable oil or oil spray for frying

1 Place all of the pancake ingredients in a liquidiser or food processor and blend until smooth.

2 Alternatively, mix the flours in a bowl. Make a well in the centre. Beat the egg and milk and gradually add to the flour, beating to make a smooth batter.

3 Place a non-stick frying pan over a high heat. Spray with oil spray or add a few drops of oil.

4 Pour in enough batter to coat the pan thinly and cook for 1–2 minutes until golden brown on the underside.

5 Turn the pancake and cook the other side for 30–60 seconds.

6 Turn out on a plate, cover and keep warm while you make the other pancakes.

7 Serve with any of the fillings below.

Pancake fillings:

- lemon juice and sugar
- sliced banana mixed with a little honey
- sliced strawberries mixed with strawberry fromage frais
- apple purée and sultanas
- raspberries, lightly mashed with a little sugar
- frozen summer fruit mixture (thawed)
- sliced mango
- tinned pineapple
- sliced fresh or tinned apricots mixed with a little apricot yoghurt
- mixed berry fruits
- tinned cherries mixed with a little greek yoghurt
- sliced fresh nectarines or peaches

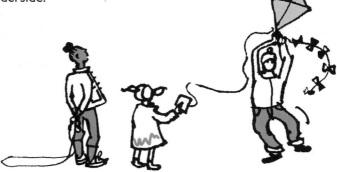

CRUNCHY APPLE CRUMBLE

This is a delicious way of adding extra fruit to your children's diet. The wholemeal flour provides iron, fibre and B vitamins, and the almonds provide protein and calcium.

Makes 4 servings

Filling
700 g (1½ lb) cooking apples, peeled and sliced
60 g (2 oz) raisins
40 g (1½ oz) sugar
½ tsp cinnamon
4 tbsp (60 ml) water
Topping
60 g (2 oz) plain flour
60 g (2 oz) wholemeal flour
60 g (2 oz) butter or margarine
40 g (1½ oz) brown sugar
25 g (1 oz) toasted almonds, chopped (or walnuts, pecans or hazelnuts)

1 Preheat the oven to 190°C/ 375°C/ gas mark 5.
2 Place the apples, raisins, sugar and cinnamon in a deep baking dish. Combine well and pour the water over.
3 For the topping, put the flour in a bowl and rub in the butter until the mixture resembles coarse breadcrumbs. Mix in the sugar and almonds.
4 Sprinkle over the apples. Bake for 20–25 minutes.

Variations

Substitute 700 g (1½ lb) prepared fruit for the apples. Try the following:
- apples and blackberries
- chopped rhubarb and sugar
- fresh or tinned apricots
- pears and raspberries
- fresh plums
- gooseberries
- pears and bananas

BAKED RICE PUDDING

This is a great-tasting nutritious pudding, simple to make and far superior to the tinned variety. It's rich in calcium and protein. Top with fresh fruit or fruit purée.

Makes 4 servings

3 tbsp (45 ml) pudding rice
600 ml (1 pint) milk (full-fat or semi-skimmed)
40 g (1½ oz) sugar
Grated nutmeg

1 Pre-heat the oven to 150°C/ 300°F/ gas mark 2.
2 Put the rice, milk and sugar in a 1.8 l (3 pint) pie dish. Stir the mixture, then grate over the nutmeg.
3 Bake for 1½ hours or until the milk has been absorbed and there is a light brown skin on top of the pudding.
4 Serve with any of the following:
- ready-made fruit compote
- stewed apples
- sliced peaches or nectarines
- stewed plums
- fresh raspberries, blueberries or blackberries

BANANA BREAD PUDDING

This pudding is warming and comforting, great for cold days! It provides carbohydrate, fibre, protein and calcium. You can substitute raisins or stewed plums for the bananas—delicious!

Makes 4 servings

6 large slices wholemeal bread
40 g (1½ oz) butter
2 small bananas, sliced
40 g (1½ oz) sugar
2 size 3 eggs
400 ml (14 fl oz) milk (full-fat or semi-skimmed)
Ground cinnamon

1 Pre-heat the oven to 180°C/ 350°F/ gas mark 4.
2 Trim the crusts from the bread, spread lightly with butter and cut into quarters diagonally.
3 Arrange one third of the bread triangles in a lightly oiled baking dish.
4 Arrange one of the sliced bananas on top and repeat the layers, finishing with the bread.
5 Combine the sugar, eggs, and milk. Pour over the bread then sprinkle with cinnamon.
6 If you have time, allow to stand for 30 minutes.
7 Bake for 40 minutes until the pudding is set and golden brown.

BAKED BANANAS

This is one of the easiest desserts. It is high in carbohydrate, low in fat, rich in potassium and magnesium.

Makes 4 servings

4 bananas
4 tbsp (60 ml) water
2 tbsp (30 ml) clear honey or maple syrup
½ teaspoon (2.5 ml) mixed spice
40 g (1½ oz) raisins

1 Preheat the oven to 200°C/ 400°F/ gas mark 6.
2 Chop the bananas into 2.5 cm (1 in) chunks.
3 Place in a baking dish and combine with the remaining ingredients.
4 Bake for 15 minutes. Serve with plain yoghurt, greek yoghurt or fromage frais.

YOGHURT AND FRUIT PUDDING

A nutritious everyday pudding that counts towards the 5 servings of fruit or vegetables recommended for children.

Makes 1 serving

1 carton (125 g or 150 g) fruit yoghurt
125 g (4 oz) fresh or stewed fruit e.g. mango, strawberries, blueberries, raspberries, peaches, bananas
1 tbsp (15 ml) toasted flaked almonds (or hazelnuts)

1 Spoon half of the yoghurt into a sundae glass (or small dish).
2 Top with half of the fruit followed by another layer of yoghurt.
3 Top with the remaining fruit and nuts.

CHERRY CLAFOUTI

This baked French custard is low in fat and a good source of protein, vitamins and calcium. You can substitute other fresh or tinned fruit, such as apricots, prunes, plums or pears for the cherries.

Makes 4 servings

60 g (2 oz) plain flour
60 g (2 oz) sugar
2 size 3 eggs
350 ml (12 fl oz) milk
1 tin (400 g) black cherries
Pinch of grated nutmeg
A little sunflower oil

1 Pre-heat the oven to 200°C/ 400°F/ gas mark 6. Lightly oil a shallow baking dish with sunflower oil.

2 Blend the flour, sugar, eggs and milk in a liquidiser.

3 Arrange the cherries evenly in the bottom of the baking dish.

4 Pour in the batter and sprinkle the top with nutmeg.

5 Bake for 40–45 minutes until the custard is firm.

BANANA AND NUT FOOL

This creamy pudding is a great source of protein, calcium and potassium.

Makes 4 servings

2 bananas
Juice of ½ lemon
150 g (5 oz) 'thick and creamy' yoghurt or Greek yoghurt
60 g (2 oz) chopped nuts, e.g. walnuts, pistachios

1 Mash the bananas with a fork and combine with the lemon juice.

2 Stir in the yoghurt and nuts and spoon into 4 bowls.

SUMMER FRUIT SALAD 1

Try to combine fruits with contrasting colours. This helps to make it more appealing to children. Remember, all types of berries (strawberries, raspberries, blackcurrants, blackberries, blueberries) are rich in vitamin C. Orange-coloured fruit, such as cantaloupe melon, apricots and nectarines are rich in beta-carotene. And the more intensely coloured the fruit, the better the antioxidant content.

Makes 4 servings

125 g (4 oz) strawberries
4 slices cantaloupe melon, diced
1 nectarine, chopped
200 ml (7 fl oz) unsweetened fruit juice, e.g. pineapple, orange, orange & mango

1 Combine the prepared fruit and fruit juice in a bowl.

2 Spoon into individual bowls and serve with fromage frais.

SUMMER FRUIT SALAD 2

225 g (8 oz) raspberries
225 g (8 oz) green grapes
200 ml (7 fl oz) apple juice

1 Combine the prepared fruit and fruit juice in a bowl.

2 Spoon into individual bowls and serve with fromage frais.

WINTER FRUIT SALAD

Make the most of vitamin C-rich citrus fruit by combining with other seasonal fruits such as apples and pears.

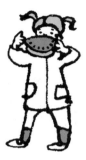

Makes 4 servings

1 apple, thinly sliced
2 clementines
2 kiwi fruit, peeled and sliced
200 ml (7 fl oz) orange juice

1 Combine the prepared fruit and fruit juice in a bowl.

2 Spoon into individual bowls and serve with fromage frais.

20 KIDS' SNACKS

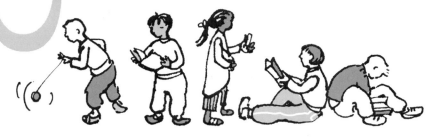

HUMMUS

Hummus makes a great snack. Serve as a dip with crudités to encourage children to eat more vegetables. It also makes a satisfying sandwich filling or jacket potato topping.

Makes about 600 ml (1 pint)

225 g (8 oz) chickpeas, soaked
overnight (or 2 tins (800 g))
2 garlic cloves
2 tbsp (30 ml) olive oil
4 tbsp (60 ml) tahini
Juice of 1 lemon
Pinch of paprika
Freshly ground black pepper

1 If using dried chickpeas drain then cook in plenty of water for about 60–90 mins or according to directions on the packet. Drain, reserving the liquid. For tinned chickpeas drain and rinse, reserving the liquid.

2 Purée the cooked or tinned chickpeas with the remaining ingredients with enough of the cooking liquid or juice from the tin to make a creamy consistency.

3 Taste and add more black pepper or lemon juice if necessary.

4 Chill in the fridge.

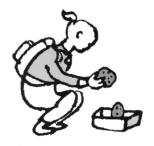

APPLE MUFFINS

These healthy muffins are excellent for lunch boxes and after-school snacks. The apples boost the fibre and vitamin content of the muffins.

Makes 12 muffins

60 ml (2 fl oz) sunflower oil
125 g (4 oz) soft brown sugar
2 size 3 eggs
125 ml (4 fl oz) milk (full-fat or semi-skimmed)
1 tsp (5 ml) vanilla extract
2 apples, peeled, cored and grated
225 g (8 oz) self-raising flour

1 Pre-heat the oven to 190°C/ 375°F/ gas mark 5.
2 Combine the oil, sugar, eggs, milk and vanilla extract in a bowl.
3 Stir in the grated apples and flour.
4 Spoon the mixture into non-stick muffin tins. Bake for 15–20 minutes until golden brown.

FRUIT MUFFINS

These are perfect refuelling snacks after sport. They are made with wholemeal flour, which is rich in fibre, iron, B vitamins and raisins, a great source of antioxidants. Make sure you pop one in your children's kit bags.

Makes 12 muffins

125 g (4 oz) white self-raising flour
125 g (4 oz) wholemeal self-raising flour
Pinch of salt
40 g (1½ oz) soft brown sugar
2 tbsp (30 ml) rapeseed oil
1 size 3 egg
200 ml (7 fl oz) milk
85 g (3 oz) raisins or sultanas

1 Pre-heat the oven to 220°C/ 425°F/ gas mark 7.
2 Mix the flours and salt together in a bowl.
3 Add the sugar, oil, egg and milk. Mix well.
4 Stir in the dried fruit.
5 Spoon into non-stick muffin tins and bake for 15–20 minutes until golden brown.

BANANA MUFFINS

These more-ish banana muffins make great after-sport or after-school snacks.

Makes 12 muffins

2 large ripe bananas, mashed
85 g (3 oz) soft brown sugar
4 tbsp (60 ml) rapeseed oil
1 size 3 egg
125 ml (4 fl oz) milk
200 g (7 oz) self-raising flour
Pinch of salt
½ tsp (2.5 ml) nutmeg, grated

1 Preheat the oven to 190°C/ 375°F/ gas mark 5.
2 In a bowl, mix together the bananas, sugar and oil.
3 Beat in the egg and milk.
4 Fold in the flour, salt and nutmeg.
5 Spoon into non-stick muffin tins and bake for 15–20 minutes.

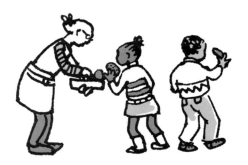

BANANA LOAF

This popular cake is made with wholemeal flour, brown sugar and rapeseed oil, instead of the usual white flour, white sugar and butter.

Makes 12 slices

225 g (8 oz) self-raising wholemeal flour
125 g (4 oz) brown sugar
Pinch of salt
½ teaspoon each of mixed spice and cinnamon
2 large ripe bananas
175 ml (6 fl oz) orange juice
2 size 3 eggs
4 tbsp (60 ml) rapeseed oil

1 Pre-heat the oven to 170°C/ 325°F/ gas mark 4.
2 Mix together the flour, sugar, salt and spices in a bowl.
3 Mash the bananas with the orange juice.
4 Combine the mashed banana mixture, eggs and oil with the flour mixture.
5 Spoon into a lightly oiled 2 lb loaf tin.
6 Bake for about 1 hour. Check the cake is done by inserting a skewer or knife into the centre. It should come out clean.

APPLE SPICE CAKE

This recipe is a great way of adding extra fruit to your children's diet. The grated apple and the rapeseed oil make this cake deliciously moist.

Makes 12 slices

300 g (10 oz) self-raising flour (half wholemeal, half white)
125 g (4 oz) brown sugar
1 tsp (5 ml) cinnamon
2 cooking apples, peeled and grated
4 tbsp (60 ml) rapeseed oil
2 size 3 eggs
125 ml (4 fl oz) milk

1 Preheat the oven to 170°C/ 325°F/ gas mark 4.

2 Mix together the flour, sugar and cinnamon in a bowl.

3 Add the grated apple, rapeseed oil, eggs and milk and combine well.

4 Spoon into a lightly oiled loaf tin and bake for about 1–1¼ hours. Check the cake is done by inserting a skewer or knife into the centre. It should come out clean.

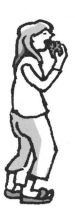

CARROT CAKE

Traditional carrot cakes have a very high oil/fat and sugar content and are smothered in cream cheese. This version is lower in fat and sugar, and is made with grated apples and carrots.

Makes 16 slices

225 g (8 oz) self-raising flour (half wholemeal, half white)
Pinch of salt
1 tsp (5ml) cinnamon
1 tsp (5 ml) nutmeg
125 g (4 oz) brown sugar
2 size 3 eggs
1 tsp (5 ml) vanilla extract
3 carrots, grated
2 apples, grated
4 tbsp (60 ml) rapeseed oil
125 ml (4 fl oz) milk

1 Pre-heat the oven to 170°C/ 325°F/ gas mark 4.

2 Mix together the flour, salt, spices and sugar in a bowl.

3 Stir in the eggs, vanilla, carrots, apples, oil and milk.

4 Line a loaf tin or a 20 cm (8 in) round cake tin with greaseproof paper. Spoon in the cake mixture.

5 Bake for about 1 hour. Check that the cake is done by inserting a skewer or knife into the centre. It should come out clean.

FRUIT CAKE

The dried fruit and grated apple add plenty of vitamins and fibre to this cake. It makes a nutritious snack anytime.

Makes 16 slices

225 g (8 oz) self-raising flour
85 g (3 oz) brown sugar
1 tsp (5 ml) cinnamon
2 size 3 eggs
4 tbsp (60 ml) rapeseed oil
1 tsp (5 ml) vanilla extract
225 g (8 oz) dried fruit mixture
1 apple, grated
85 ml (3 fl oz) milk

1 Pre-heat the oven to 170°C/ 325°F/ gas mark 4.

2 Mix together the flour, sugar and cinnamon in a bowl.

3 Make a well in the centre and add the eggs, oil, vanilla, dried fruit, apple and milk. Combine together well.

4 Spoon into a 20 cm (8 in) round or square baking tin and bake for about 1¼–1½ hours. Check the cake is done by inserting a skewer or knife into the centre. It should come out clean.

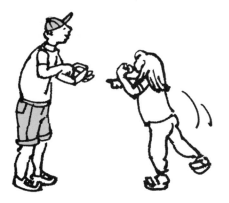

GINGER SPICE CAKE

This delicious cake is lower in fat and sugar than the traditional version, yet is deliciously moist as it is made with rapeseed oil, which is rich in healthy monounsaturates.

Makes 10 slices

200 g (7 oz) plain flour
1 tsp (5 ml) bicarbonate of soda
1 tsp (5 ml) cinnamon
1 tsp (5 ml) ginger
1 tsp (5 ml) ground cloves
1 size 3 egg
125 g (4 oz) soft brown sugar
4 tbsp (60 ml) rapeseed oil
200 ml (7 oz) low-fat plain yoghurt
1 tbsp (15 ml) Demerara sugar
1 tbsp (115 ml) pecan nuts, chopped

1 Pre-heat the oven to 170°C/ 325°F/ gas mark 3.

2 Lightly oil a 1.5 l (2½ pint) loaf tin.

3 Place the flour, bicarbonate of soda and spices in a bowl and mix together.

4 Whisk the egg, sugar and oil together until light and fluffy. Stir in the low-fat yoghurt and mix well.

5 Gently fold in the flour and spice mixture.

6 Spoon into the prepared tin and sprinkle with the Demerara sugar and chopped nuts.

7 Bake for 45 minutes. Check the cake is done by inserting a skewer or knife into the centre. It should come out clean. Allow to cool for a few minutes before turning out on to a cooling rack.

WHOLEMEAL RAISIN BISCUITS

These biscuits are far healthier than bought ones. They are lower in sugar and higher in fibre.

Makes 20 biscuits

225 g (8 oz) wholemeal plain flour
40 g (1½ oz) brown sugar
85 g (3 oz) raisins
2 tbsp (30 ml) rapeseed oil
1 size 3 egg
4 tbsp (60 ml) milk

1 Preheat the oven to 180°C/ 350°F/ gas mark 4.
2 Combine the flour, sugar and raisins in a bowl.
3 Stir in the oil, egg and milk and lightly mix together until you have a stiff dough.
4 Place spoonfuls of the mixture onto a lightly oiled baking tray.
5 Bake for 12–15 minutes until golden brown.

APRICOT BARS

Dried apricots are packed with beta-carotene, a powerful antioxidant that's also good for the skin.

Makes 8 bars

125 g (4 oz) self-raising white flour
60 g (2 oz) sugar
125 g (4 oz) dried apricots
6 tbsp (90 ml) orange juice
2 size 3 eggs
125 g (4 oz) sultanas

1 Preheat the oven to 180°C/ 350°F/ gas mark 4.
2 Mix together the flour and sugar in a bowl.
3 Blend together the apricots and juice in a liquidiser or food processor until smooth.
4 Add the apricot purée, eggs and sultanas to the flour & sugar. Mix together.
5 Spoon the mixture into an 18 cm (7 in) square cake tin. Bake at for 30–35 minutes until golden brown. Allow to cool. Cut into 8 bars.

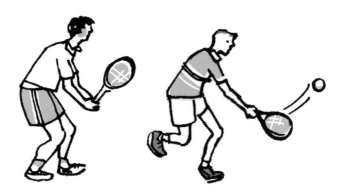

CEREAL BARS

These highly nutritious bars are made from oats and muesli, which provide slow-release sustained energy. They are lower in fat than commercial cereal bars.

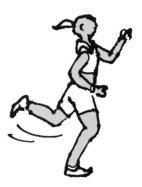

Makes 12 bars

175 g (6 oz) oats
85 g (3 oz) no added sugar muesli
150 g (5 oz) dried fruit mixture
3 tbsp (45 ml) honey, clear or set
2 egg whites
175 ml (6 fl oz) apple juice

1 Pre-heat the oven to 180°C/ 350°F/ gas mark 4.
2 Combine the oats, muesli and dried fruit in a bowl.
3 Warm the honey in a small saucepan until it is runny. Add to the bowl.
4 Stir in the remaining ingredients.
5 Press the mixture into a lightly oiled 18 × 28 cm (7 × 11 in) baking tin. Bake for 20–25 minutes until golden. When cool, cut into bars.

21 DELICIOUS DRINKS

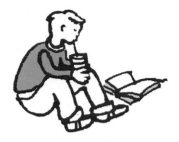

BANANA MILKSHAKE

This simple, nutritious shake makes a great refu-elling drink at any time of the day.

Makes 2 servings
250 ml (8 fl oz) milk (full-fat or semi-skimmed)
2 ripe bananas, sliced
Few ice cubes, crushed

- Put the milk, crushed ice and banana in a blender. Blend until smooth, thick and bubbly.

STRAWBERRY MILKSHAKE

Strawberries are an excellent source of vitamin C.

Makes 2 servings
150 ml (¼ pint) milk (full-fat or semi-skimmed)
1 × 125 g carton low-fat strawberry yoghurt
1 handful of strawberries
Few ice cubes, crushed

- Put the milk, crushed ice and strawberries in a blender. Blend until smooth, thick and bubbly.

BANANA SMOOTHIE

This velvet-thick smoothie is made simply from fruit and yoghurt, and doubles as a nourishing dessert.

Makes 2 servings
1 large ripe banana
1 carton (150 g) plain bio-yoghurt
2 tsp (10 ml) honey
60 ml (2 fl oz) apple juice

- Blend all the ingredients in a liquidiser then serve.

MANGO AND STRAWBERRY SMOOTHIE

Mangoes are a terrific source of beta-carotene, while strawberries provide lots of vitamin C. A super nutritious drink!

Makes 2 servings
1 small mango
125 g (4 oz) strawberries
1 banana
200 ml (7 fl oz) apple juice

1 Peel the banana and peel and stone the mango. Place all the fruit in a blender and blend until smooth.

2 Add the apple juice and blend for a few more seconds. If you wish, you can reduce the quantity of juice to give a thicker drink.

BERRY CRUSH

This drink is bursting with vitamin C and cancer-protective phytochemicals.

Makes 2 servings
225 g (8 oz) mixture of fresh or frozen berries, e.g. raspberries, blueberries, strawberries, blackcurrants
1 carton (150 g) raspberry bio-yoghurt
200 ml (7 fl oz) milk (full-fat or semi-skimmed)

• Put all the ingredients in a blender and blend until smooth.

TROPICAL DELIGHT

The mango and papaya provide lots of beta-carotene and the lime juice is rich in vitamin C.

Makes 2 servings
1 mango, peeled and stoned
4 slices fresh or tinned pineapple
1 papaya, peeled and de-seeded
Juice of 1 lime
Ice cubes

• Put the fruit and ice in a blender and blend until smooth.

ENERGISER

Here's a smoothie that's full of beta-carotene, vitamin C and potassium. It is a great energiser and immune booster.

Makes 2 servings
1 banana
1 peach
125 g (4 oz) raspberries (or strawberries)
125 ml (4 fl oz) orange juice

• Place all the fruit and the orange juice in a blender and blend until smooth.

STRAWBERRY AND BANANA MILKSHAKE

Banana and strawberries make a delicious combination. This nutritious drink makes a great after-school or post-exercise drink.

Makes 2 servings

1 banana
125 g (4 oz) strawberries
1 carton (150 g) strawberry bio-yoghurt
120 ml (4 fl oz) milk (full-fat or semi-skimmed)

- Place the fruit, yoghurt and milk in a blender and blend until smooth.

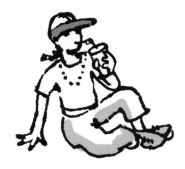

ON-LINE RESOURCES

www.kidshealth   Offers health, nutrition and fitness advice for
                                      parents, kids and teenagers.

www.eatright.org   The website of the American Dietetic
                                      Association, gives nutrition news, tips and
                                      resources.

www.nutrition.org.uk   The website of the British Nutrition Foundation,
                                      gives information, news and educational
                                      resources.

www.nutrio.com   Includes a useful section on kids' nutrition.

www.edauk.com   The website of the Eating Disorders Association,
                                      offering information and help on all aspects of
                                      eating disorders.

www.eating-disorders.com   The website of the US Center for Eating
                                      Disorders, offers information and support.

www.USDA.gov   Includes a section on children's nutrition.

USEFUL ADDRESSES

Eating Disorders Association   First Floor, Wensum House, 103 Prince of Wales
                                      Road, Norwich, NR1 1DW
                                      Youth help line (18 years and under):
                                      01603 765050 (4–6 pm Monday–Friday).
                                      Telephone help line: 01603 621414 (9 am–6.30 pm
                                      Monday–Friday)

British Nutrition Foundation   52–54 High Holborn, London WC1V 6RQ

FURTHER READING

Anorexia Nervosa: A Survival Guide for Families, Friends and Sufferers
Treasure, J. (1997) Psychology Press.

Anorexia Nervosa: The Wish to Change: A Self-Help Guide
Crisp, A. H. *et al* (1996) Psychology Press.

Eating Disorders: A Parents' Guide
Bryant-Waugh, R. and Lask, B. (1999) Penguin.

Quick Children's Meals
Karmel, A. (1997) Ebury Press.

Super Foods for Children
Van Straten, M. and Griggs, B. (2001) Dorling Kindersley.

The Food Our Children Eat
Blythman, J. (1999) Fourth Estate.

The Young Athlete's Handbook
Youth Sport Trust (2001) Human Kinetics.

REFERENCES

Page

4   Gregory, J. *et al.* (2000) *National Diet and Nutrition Survey: young people aged 4 to 18 years. Volume 1: Report of the National Diet and Nutrition Survey.* The Stationery Office.

5   Tounian, P., 'Presence of increased stiffness of the common carotid artery and endothelial dysfunction in severely obese children: a prospective study.' *The Lancet*, 358 (2001) 1400.
     Consumers International (1996) *A Spoonful of Sugar—Television food advertising aimed at children; an international comparative study.*
     The Food Commission, 'Sweet Persuasion'. *The Food Magazine*, 9 (1990).
     The Food Commission, 'A Diet of Junk Food Adverts'. II, (1992) 11.

6   National Food Alliance (1996) *Easy to swallow, hard to stomach: the results of a survey of food advertising on television.*

Which? December 2001.

9 Organix (2002) *Carrot or Chemistry*. Organix Brands.

The Food Commission (2000) Report, *Children's Food Examined*. Food Commission.

The Food Commission (2000) *The Food Commission's Guide to Children's Food*. Food Commission.

32 Leeds A., Brand Miller, J., Foster-Powell K. and Colagiuri, S. (2000) *The Glucose Revolution*. Hodder & Stoughton.

McCance & Widdowson (1991) *The Composition of Foods*, 5th edn. MAFF/ RSC. CompEat 5 software. Nutrition Systems: Grantham.

54 Prior, R. L., and Cao, G. (2000) 'Analysis of botanicals and dietary supplements for antioxidant capacity: a review.' *Journal of AOAC International*, 83(4) 950–6.

77 Cole, T. J., Bellizzi, M., Flegal, K. and Dietz W. H. (2000) 'Establishing a standard definition for child overweight and obesity worldwide: international survey.' *British Medical Journal*, 320: 1240.

Reilly, J. J., Dorosty, A. R, and Emmett, P. M. (1999) 'Prevalence of overweight and obesity in British children: cohort study.' *British Medical Journal*, 319: 1039.

Rudolf, M. C. J. *et al.* (2001) 'Increasing prevalence of obesity in primary school children: cohort study.' *British Medical Journal*, 322: 1094–5.

79 Burke, V. *et al.* (2001) 'Family lifestyle and parental body mass index as predictors of body mass index in Australian children: a longitudinal study.' *International Journal of Obesity*, 25: 147–57.

Lake, J. K., Power, C. and Cole, T. J. (1997) 'Child to adult body mass index in the 1958 British birth cohort: associations with parental obesity.' *Archive of Diseases in Childhood*, 77(5): 376–81.

81 Bouchard, C. (1992) 'Genetic aspects of human obesity.' In *Obesity*, P. Bjornthorp and B. N. Brodoff (eds) J. P. Lippincott, 343–51.

98 Dowshen, S. (2001) 'Strength training and your child,' *www.KidsHealth.com*.

102 Gardner Merchant (1996) *The Gardner Merchant Schools Meals Survey: What Are Our Children Eating?* Kenley: Gardner Merchant.

109 Caroline Walker Trust (1992) *Nutritional Guidelines for School Meals*. Caroline Walker Trust, or *www.dfee.gov.uk/schoollunches*.

114 Sungot-Borgon, J. (1994) 'Eating disorders in female athletes.' *British Journal of Sports Medicine*, 17(3) 176–88.

INDEX

Page numbers in bold = recipe

Other titles by Anita Bean:

- The Complete Guide to Strength Training
- The Complete Guide to Sports Nutrition
- Food for Fitness

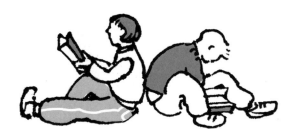